Everyday Mobility and Health

SCIENCES

*Geography and Demography*, Field Director – Denise Pumain

*Infrastructure and Mobility Networks Geography*,
Subject Heads – Hadrien Commenges and Florent Le Néchet

# Everyday Mobility and Health

*Coordinated by*
Julie Vallée

iSTE

WILEY

First published 2024 in Great Britain and the United States by ISTE Ltd and John Wiley & Sons, Inc.



ISTE Ltd
27-37 St George's Road
London SW19 4EU
UK

www.iste.co.uk

John Wiley & Sons, Inc.
111 River Street
Hoboken, NJ 07030
USA

www.wiley.com



Library of Congress Control Number: 2023949778

British Library Cataloguing-in-Publication Data
A CIP record for this book is available from the British Library
ISBN 978-1-78945-109-2

ERC code:
SH2 Institutions, Values, Environment and Space
*SH2_8 Energy, transportation and mobility*
*SH2_11 Human, economic and social geography*
SH3 The Social World, Diversity, Population
*SH3_9 Health, ageing and society*

# Contents

# Introduction

**Julie VALLÉE**
*Géographie-cités, CNRS, Paris, France*

## From the individual to the geographical space

In the field of health, the daily mobility of individuals can be considered through the lens of the advantages it provides (reduction of social isolation, access to services and equipment far from places of residence, physical activity, etc.), or in terms of the inconveniences it causes (exposure to pollution, traffic accidents, strenuous commuting, etc.). On the contrary, we can also analyze the way in which the physical and mental health of an individual promotes or hinders their daily travels, whether in terms of the distance covered or the availability of modes of transport, and how these are actually used. These different approaches focus on the individual as the entry and exit point; the challenge is to study the influence of the individual's daily mobility on health, as well as the influence of the individual's health on mobility.

However, this relationship between everyday mobility and health does not take place at the level of independent individuals: the daily mobility of some people has an impact on the daily mobility of others (e.g. traffic jams can lead some individuals to shift their departure time, to modify their journey or to change their modes of transport), whereas the health of some people has an impact on the health of others (by contagion effect). Therefore, both mobility and health are the product of the interactions between individuals. But individuals are not the only actors involved in this system: social and political structures are also present. Public actors organize the mobility and healthcare provision throughout the local and national territory and promote their uses among individuals. Not only do social structures affect the mobility and health behaviors of individuals, but also public health and regional planning policies.

The role of geographical space within this system is multifaceted: it influences the daily mobility of individuals through the transport system and the built environment. Depending on geographical places, people's living conditions may vary, together with the local health norms or the availability and quality of the healthcare provision. It would nonetheless be simplistic to imagine that geographical space has a compartmentalized impact on people's daily mobility, on the one hand, and on their health, on the other hand. In fact, it is the geographical space that structures their relationship. To illustrate this mechanism, we can observe that the distribution of the healthcare provision throughout the territory is not independent from the mobility of individuals, or that the trips of some transform the quality of the living environments of others, and as such, their health.

## Organization of the book

Without claiming to exhaust the richness and complexity of the subject, the purpose of this work is to present the different aspects of the relationship between everyday mobility and health, taking into account the social, political and geographical components of the system in which this relationship thrives. This book is made up of seven chapters structured into three main parts.

*Part 1* is devoted to the diffusion and exposure mechanisms related to the daily mobility of individuals. *Chapter 1*, written by Alexandre Cebeillac and Éric Daudé, illustrates how daily mobility – which modifies the exposure of individuals to pathogens – renews research on the spatial and temporal diffusion of communicable diseases. *Chapter 2*, written by Camille Perchoux, presents the methodological issues related to taking into account people's daily mobility when measuring environmental effects on health. These first two chapters complement one another: they discuss the methodological issues relating to the consideration of everyday mobility in the diffusion of health problems within the geographical space and in the exposure of individuals to geographical spaces. *Chapter 3*, written by Martine Shareck, also addresses the exposure of individuals to the environment, but specifically calls into question the social inequalities that socially differentiated mobility induces in terms of exposure and health.

*Part 2* is dedicated to daily environments and active transportation (mainly walking and cycling) at a time when this trend is generating great interest: on the one hand, because it induces increased physical expenditure (and in this way can reduce the risk of obesity and associated chronic pathologies), and on the other hand, because it limits the carbon emissions from car travel, contributing to the fight against global warming. The use of active transportation is eased (or hindered) by certain local characteristics of the built environment (see the notions of walkability and bikeability), which will be detailed and discussed in the fourth and fifth chapters of this book. *Chapter 4*, co-written by Marie-Soleil Cloutier and Karine Lachapelle, specifically addresses walking and insists on the various sources of insecurity that pedestrians may encounter in the geographical space. In *Chapter 5*, Thierry Feuillet and Hélène Charreire revisit the local contexts that are more or less favorable to active transportation, with a special focus on the territorial heterogeneity of relationships between the living environment and active mobility. These two chapters present several interventions intended to promote (and secure) the use of active transportation and discuss the difficulty in evaluating the effectiveness of such experiments.

Addressed by the two previous chapters in connection with active mobility, the question of policies – and the place they give to daily mobility – is at the heart of *Part 3* of the book. *Chapter 6*, written by Stephanie Alexander, offers a critical analysis of the actions and policies that promote physical activity and active mobility by detailing their underlying assumptions and values around public health. *Chapter 7*, co-authored by Véronique Lucas-Gabrielli and Catherine Mangeney, discusses the role of daily mobility in the policies for rationalizing the healthcare provision. It presents the way in which everyday mobility is taken into account in measures of spatial accessibility to healthcare and in the delimitation of priority areas with insufficient healthcare provision.

Following this three-part structure is only a key to reading the book. The seven chapters can also be read according to the health indicators considered, the ways of analyzing daily mobility, the mechanisms involving the geographical space and the living environments or the challenges (methodological, political or contemporary) raised and debated (see Table I.1).

| Part | 1 | | | 2 | | 3 | |
|---|---|---|---|---|---|---|---|
| **Chapter** | **1** | **2** | **3** | **4** | **5** | **6** | **7** |
| **Health indicators** | | | | | | | |
| Communicable diseases | • | | | | | | |
| Obesity (and associated chronic diseases) | | | | | • | • | |
| Road accidents | | | | • | | | |
| Access to healthcare | | | | | | | • |
| Diverse and varied indicators | | • | • | | | | |
| **Ways to analyze daily mobility** | | | | | | | |
| Spatio-temporal dynamics | • | | | | | | |
| Activity space | | • | • | | | | |
| Social and spatial justice | | | • | | | | • |
| Accessibility to services | | • | • | | | | • |
| Injunctions; constrained versus chosen mobility | | • | • | | | • | |
| Benefits and risks associated with active mobility | | | | • | • | • | |
| **Geographical space and the living environments…** | | | | | | | |
| in which pathogens spread | • | | | | | | |
| to which individuals are exposed | • | • | • | • | • | | • |
| where the services are localized | | • | • | | | | • |
| favorable to active mobility | | | | • | • | • | |
| **Challenges…** | | | | | | | |
| in methodology (data and measures) | • | • | • | | • | | • |
| for regional planning | | | | • | • | | • |
| for public health | • | • | • | • | • | • | • |
| of today's world (Covid-19…) | • | | • | | • | • | |

**Table I.1.** *Synthesis of the themes developed in the seven chapters of the book*

# PART 1

# Diffusion and Exposure Mechanisms Related to Daily Mobility

# 1

# Daily Mobility and the Spread of Communicable Infectious Diseases

**Alexandre CEBEILLAC**[1,2] **and Eric DAUDÉ**[1]
*1 IDEES, CNRS, Normandie Université, Rouen, France*
*2 Institut Pasteur, Paris, France*

## 1.1. Introduction

Communicable infectious diseases are caused by microorganisms, called pathogens (viruses, fungi, bacteria, parasites) that infect a living organism, called the host. Pathogens are transmitted from an infected host to a healthy host through various channels. A first category of transmission channels involves direct, physical contact (saliva, blood, sexual contact: AIDS, hepatitis B, syphilis, etc.) or the air or respiratory tract (cough: flu, tuberculosis, pertussis, nasopharyngitis, etc.). A second category involves an indirect mode of transmission, either by ingestion (food, water: hepatitis A, cholera, rotavirus, poliomyelitis) or through a vector (mosquito, tick, flea: dengue fever, Zika, Chikungunya, Lyme). Whether direct or indirect, this transmission pattern implies the proximity of hosts moving around the same geographic space. Mobility therefore becomes a key element for understanding the spread of epidemics.

---

For a color version of all the figures in this chapter, see www.iste.co.uk/vallee/everyday.zip.

*Everyday Mobility and Health*,
coordinated by Julie VALLÉE. 

An epidemic corresponds to a rapid increase in the number of cases of a disease in a local or national area – a pandemic is its global expression. Identifying the emergence of the pathogen responsible for a disease as well as its modes of propagation should enable a better understanding, or even anticipation, of its geographical diffusion. The example of the spread of Covid-19 after the first cases were identified in China evidences the weight of international (and then national) mobility in this propagation. At a local scale, in everyday spaces, the role and weight of mobility is more complex to disentangle, because mobility is concomitant with many other factors which, combined, lead to local disease diffusion mappings: local disease surveillance and control actions, characteristics of the environments visited, behavior of the populations at risk, etc. This complexity partly explains why local daily mobility has long remained understudied in retrospective analyses. In the majority of cases, individual exposure factors are solely deduced from the characteristics of the living space of sick people, a bias partly related to the recording of the case at their place of residence. However, this obstacle tends to be partially surmounted thanks to digital tools and data. As it modifies a static vision of the exposure to pathogens, daily mobility renews research on the spread of communicable diseases.

The first section of this chapter (section 1.2) will summarize the evolution of knowledge on the contagiousness of diseases and their modes of transmission in an epidemic context, emphasizing the link between daily mobility and epidemiology. The modeling of daily mobility will be addressed in section 1.3. We will discuss different modeling methods and the concepts used in an epidemic context. Special emphasis will be placed on the most recent classes of models, namely individual-based models (IBMs). These models integrate geographic information as well as social and epidemiological knowledge into a single formalism, enabling exploration of a wide variety of scenarios. Finally, a last section (section 1.4) will prompt a selective literature review, dedicated to the data currently in use to better understand daily mobility and to calibrate increasingly detailed epidemiological models.

## 1.2. Analyzing the role of daily mobility in the spread of epidemics: concepts, studies and tools

Understanding the mechanisms responsible for the spread of an epidemic is a prerequisite for any action attempting to prevent it. Spatial epidemiology now plays a major role in this fight.

### 1.2.1. *The path of daily mobility in the geographical reflection of infectious diseases*

When it reached Europe in 1829, little medical controversy was stirred up in identifying Asiatic cholera morbus. The symptoms described by colonial doctors stationed in India matched the symptoms observed at Europe's doorstep: "rice water" stools, profuse vomiting of liquid matter, spasms, horrible cramps, imperceptible pulse, bluish tints in the extremities and around the lips (hence the name "Blue Death"), body cooling, collapse, etc. and, above all, a mortality rate exceeding 50% in many cities. Though the poison had a name and a geographical origin, it was still necessary to determine its medical origin, its modes of propagation, the means to protect against it and the treatment to eradicate it. These questions fueled part of the medical research of the 19th century when two currents of thought collided, the insufficiency of medical knowledge leading to different interpretations of identical statistics and cartographic documents (Eliot et al. 2012).

Doctors then became divided between two schools: contagionists and anti-contagionists. In the 19th century, the sense of the term "contagion" implied that the disease was transmitted from person to person, via contact. This excluded diseases transmitted by air or water from the list of contagious diseases. One of the measures against cholera for the doctors who classified it under contagious diseases involved the isolation of any infected person in view of protecting the population: quarantine. On the other hand, anti-contagionists believed that disease was transmitted via the interactions between human beings and the environment – chiefly as a result of miasmatic exhalations. On the one hand, favorable conditions to the development and propagation of epidemics could be environment-related (climate, atmospheric density, degree of humidity, prevailing winds, the term "malaria" being derived from the Latin Mal'aria – which means "bad air" – whereas the term "palu" means a swamp) and, on the other hand, they could be owing to the type of habitat (cleanliness of houses and clothes, as well as inhabitants' mores).

Overcoming this opposition between contagionists, anti-contagionists and supporters of the miasma theory, John Snow (1813–1858) shed new light on the understanding of the modes of propagation of cholera. As Europe experienced a new epidemic onslaught and the "Blue Death" spread across the cities and the countryside, Snow identified the waterborne nature of the "poison" that was wreaking havoc from Bengal to America, and ravaging Europe.

In his famous treatise *On the Mode of Communication of Cholera* published in 1855, supplemented with maps and statistics, the English doctor offered an original demonstration to support his hypotheses on the disease's mode of propagation (Snow 1855). The singularity of Snow's work was his inclusion on medical topography maps – which occasionally recorded deaths and people contaminated by cholera – of water points by neighborhood, notably that of Broad Street in London. He proved that most of the people who died of cholera lived near dirty water points.

Apart from drawing up these maps, Snow sought to understand why certain houses in the neighborhood – for instance, the workhouse on Poland Street or the brewery on Broad Street – were spared the disease. It turned out that the former had its own water point, whereas the workers of the latter simply did not drink water because they were entitled to rations of malt[1] liquor. Another interesting fact: these surveys revealed that the deaths of certain persons living far from Broad Street were due to the fact that they preferred to drink water from this point, considering it less dirty than the source near their home[2].

When he analyzed the mortality data by gender in London in 1848, he also realized that the epidemic outbreak affected men more than women, but in time, those numbers tended to equilibrium. The interpretation – paraphrased in modern terms – is related to gender mobility trends; men having a greater ability to disperse across the city because of their work, whereas women generally stayed at home. Men had a wider variety of sources to meet their water needs and therefore, a higher risk of contamination during an epidemic outbreak. At a second stage, when cholera spread throughout the city, men and women became equally at-risk[3] populations. Snow also noted that valets and

1. "The men are allowed a certain quantity of malt liquor, and Mr. Huggins believes they do not drink water at all; and he is quite certain that the workmen never obtained water from the pump in the street" (Snow 1855).

2. "It requires to be stated that the water of the pump in Marlborough Street, at the end of Carnaby Street, was so impure that many people avoided using it. And I found that the persons who died near this pump in the beginning of September, had water from the Broad Street pump" (Snow 1855).

3. "The greater part of the female population remain almost constantly at home, and take their meals at home, whilst a considerable number of the men move about in following their occupations, and take both food and drink at a variety of places; consequently, in the early part of an epidemic, when the disease only exists in a few spots, the male part of the population is most liable to come within the operation of the morbid poison; but at a later period of the epidemic, when the cholera is more generally diffused, it may reach those who stay at home as readily as those who move about" (Snow 1855).

servants were the least affected by the disease because these workers used to live at the home of their "masters" in wealthy neighborhoods with better sanitary infrastructure. In this sense, they were affected by cholera less than their employers, whose daily routine was marked by numerous visits across the city.

The waterborne origin of cholera was thus established, as well as the first reflections on the role of mobility and the living spaces of populations, their exposure to pathogens and the spread of the epidemic. Based on these first results on cholera, Snow came to the conclusion that plague and yellow fever spread in the same way[4]. It only took a few more decades for research in epidemiology to show that both cases were vector-borne diseases. It is likely that the co-occurrence of mosquitoes with water points and the swarming of rats in slums could have misled him.

At the beginning of the 20th century, while the pathogens responsible for the main deadly diseases of the time and their mode of transmission were known, understanding the emergence and diffusion of new pathogens in epidemic form represented a challenge. This was the case of AIDS in the 1980s, of dengue in the 1990s and of SARS-CoV2 after 2019. Even if the main mechanisms contributing to the transmission and propagation of communicable diseases were known, their combinations in heterogeneous territories and within host populations with varied susceptibilities was quite complex. This required acknowledging the environmental and social criteria in which pathogens develop, the socio-demographic characteristics and behavior of hosts (in particular daily mobility and interactions) as factors of direct or indirect exposure to pathogens.

### 1.2.2. *The role of mobility in the spread of epidemics*

The spatial diffusion of an infectious and communicable disease implies that a pathogen multiplies and spreads from one host to another by means of a propagation channel (e.g. by airborne transmission or an animal vector). It is necessary to identify the actors involved in the transmission cycle (the pathogen's potential hosts and transmission channels) as well as the processes interacting within the cycle, namely the pathogen's propagation mechanisms, which lead to host contamination (Langlois and Daudé 2007).

4. In the section "Evidence that plague, yellow fever, dysentry and typhoid fever are communicated in the same way as cholera".

The *contamination process* acts on the hosts: it represents the invasion and development of the pathogen within the host. Associated with infection, this process can alter the host's health condition after the amount of pathogens present reaches a certain threshold. Different health conditions can be defined for the host, such as:

– contamination, moment of the pathogen invasion;

– infection, when the pathogen develops within the host;

– viremia or contagiousness; the period during which the host emits a sufficient amount of pathogens to contaminate another susceptible person (who has not developed immune defenses capable of fighting the infection).

These health conditions may or may not be associated with symptoms, and the infection may end in partial or total recovery, with or without immunity to the pathogen, or result in death. This process can be globally represented by the number of hosts contaminated by the pathogen and the number required to qualify the disease as an epidemic. In fact, a certain density threshold of pathogens must be reached within an individual to trigger the disease, and reach a sufficient volume of infected individuals for an epidemic to break out.

The *propagation process* represents the pathogen's "behavior" emitted from each infected host. The pathogen's survival outside the host and before the invasion of a new host depends on environmental conditions. The influenza A virus, for example, survives between one and two days on hard surfaces and less than 12 hours on fabric. We can globally represent the propagation process by the number of active pathogens in the propagation channel (in this case, the environment). When this number is very low, particularly during the pre-epidemic phase, epidemic success is a stochastic process which depends on social and environmental conditions: high concentrations of people, absence of barrier measures, unfavorable environmental conditions. This is when highly targeted control measures can prove effective for preventing the spread of the disease. Pathogen viability emitted from the infected host also depends on the behavior of its possible vector. For instance, dengue viruses transmitted by mosquitoes can pose a risk to humans throughout the infected mosquito's life cycle. When assessing epidemic risk, the number of pathogens can then be confused with the population of infected vectors.

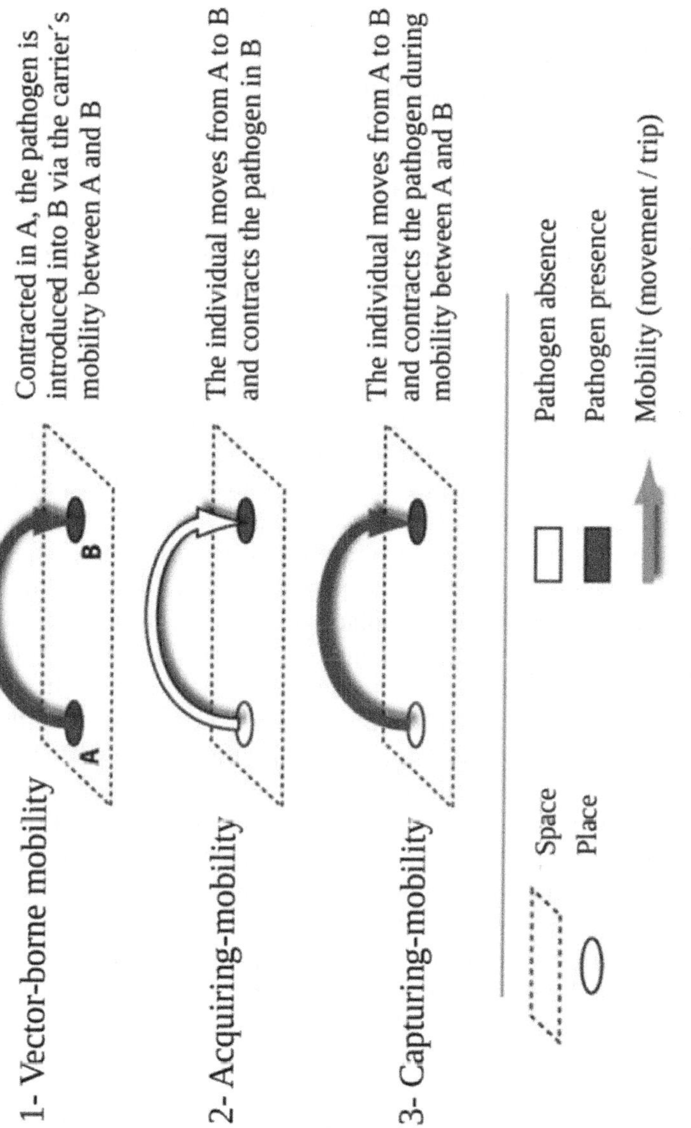


**Figure 1.1.** *Mobility and types of pathogen transmission (source: Daudé and Eliot (2005))*

By multiplying and differentiating the possible areas of contamination and propagation, the daily mobility of populations contributes to the pathogen's spatial diffusion. This offers risk reduction strategies: ceasing mobility reduces the number, nature and places for interactions between hosts and can stop – if not slow down – the spread of the disease (the intention behind quarantines and lockdowns). Knowledge about host mobility can be useful for predicting the next contamination places or for tracing contamination sources a posteriori, in view of discovering the index case (the first contaminated person). Finally, epidemiological studies in places in which populations interact (markets, schools, places of work, etc.) or in places in which hosts and vectors co-exist (gardens, parks, public transport, etc.) can be useful for identifying potential sites for the emergence of pathogens or contamination and for reducing risk at the source (school closures, vector control in gardens).

Mobility acquires a different status depending on the mechanism underlying the transmission from pathogen to host or vector. On the one hand, mobility can be an intermediary in the transmission of the infectious agent from place to place. The agent is transmitted from one place to another from an infection source (outbreak). Here, mobility is a vector of contamination (Figure 1.1, (1) "**vector-borne mobility**"). This is the case, for example, when a contagious person struck down with influenza introduces the virus into the workplace, by sharing a meal in a communal room with several susceptible colleagues. On the other hand, mobility can lead to situations featuring exposure to pathogens. In this case, contamination is the result of mobility that exposes the host through the places they frequent (Figure 1.1, (2) "**acquiring-mobility**"). Here, it is the susceptible colleague who visits the communal room at the workplace who is exposed to the pathogen, whereas at home, there was potentially no level of risk. Movement is "at the origin" of the agent's contamination. Lastly, mobility can constitute a contamination "channel". It is during transportation that the host is contaminated by a pathogen and introduces it into the place of destination, in which case we speak of "**capturing-mobility**" (Figure 1.1, (3)). This is the moment when public transport becomes a key contamination place among traveling hosts.

These three basic forms of contamination are exclusive in the propagation of a pathogen at the individual-host level, but not at the group scale, and even less so at the scale of a whole population. This makes it all the more complex to identify the most vulnerable places exposed to contamination, the riskiest journeys, the duration and number of contacts most likely to spread a given disease during trips. Field studies are a first attempt to appraise the role of these different forms of contamination underlying pathogen diffusion.

### 1.2.3. *Case studies: epidemic dynamics based on the location of proven cases*

One major difficulty when trying to assess the role and weight of daily mobility in the spread of an epidemic lies in identifying the circumstances, place and time of contamination. In the majority of cases, public health data and epidemiological surveys only identify sick people at their place of residence. Trying to reproduce the spread of the disease from clusters of patients can be misleading – a cluster of residents in a neighborhood does not necessarily convey that there is a high risk of residential contamination. By the same token, an absence of clusters based on the place of residence does not necessarily mean that another type of cluster would not have emerged if the cases had been located otherwise (e.g. at the workplace or a recreational area).

#### 1.2.3.1. *Looking for contact cases*

To overcome this limitation, further research may be conducted in order to collect ad hoc data and try to reconstruct the person's itinerary a few days or weeks prior to the illness. The search for contact cases begins with a questionnaire administered to the hospitalized or sick person to accurately trace their movements after the appearance of the first symptoms, or a few days earlier, depending on viremia. Family members, acquaintances and colleagues are also questioned in order to identify the nature and duration of contacts with the sick person.

This method varies depending on the pathogen considered, as well as its contagiousness: a highly contagious virus will require extending the field of research to the greatest number of potential contact cases, with all the inaccuracies this entails. Asking a person how long they spent near another person and at what distance at a supermarket queue systematically induces a bias which over-represents risk. Applications for detecting proximity contacts using Bluetooth technology embedded in mobile phones were developed and widely distributed during the Covid-19 pandemic to partially address this issue. Nevertheless, there is currently little feedback from experience or studies clearly defining the contributions and limitations of those methods.

### 1.2.3.2. *Spatio-temporal cluster analysis*

In addition to the monitoring of individual trajectories, spatio-temporal cluster analysis assumes that detected cases are related both in time (duration of the contagion period and exposure duration) and in space (co-presence of people during contamination). But given the fact that determining the place of contamination is difficult, these studies are often conducted taking into account the places of residence of infected people. This boundary is even more significant for vector-borne diseases, as it dissociates the co-presence of healthy and infected hosts in the contamination/propagation process. An infected host living in district A can contaminate a vector during their morning visit to a park in district B. A few days later, this same vector can contaminate a host in district B (but be living in neighborhood C) during their nightly jog. Assessing the share of contamination that occurs while traveling outside the place of residence is a real methodological challenge. Phylogeography, which studies the distribution of the different genetic lineages of a virus, is an approach that partly makes it possible to overcome this obstacle.

Viruses are organisms that tend to mutate relatively quickly, and slight mutations accompany variations in infections and transmissions. The more differences there are between two viruses affecting two people, the smaller the chances for these individuals to belong to the same contamination chain. Here lies the origin of phylogeography, a science that studies the dynamics of viruses and analyzes the evolution of their genome, producing new variants. This approach is widely used at a global scale, particularly in the context of influenza, in order to estimate which strain will be dominant and which vaccine should be recommended.

This method was used by Salje et al. (2017) to determine the contamination chains of dengue fever in Bangkok. To do this, they first developed a phylogenetic tree including 640 genetic sequences of dengue viruses, drawn from blood samples of children having suffered from dengue fever between 1994 and 2010, and whose home address was known. Two individuals belong to the same transmission chain when the differences between the genomes of the same virus are relatively small. They found that 60% of the cases in the same chain had homes less than 200 m apart, which underlines the importance of residential neighborhoods in the spread of the epidemic. Despite this, we should observe that the subjects studied by Salje et al. (2012, 2017) were children, whose mobility is narrower than that of adults, often limited to the neighborhood and to schools, in most cases, located near their homes.

In another study and with another method, Vazquez-Prokopec et al. (2010) studied the spatial distribution of homes of confirmed dengue fever cases during the 2003 epidemic, which affected the city of Cairns in Australia. It was the first major epidemic, which means that most patients had no prior experience of the virus (naïve population), and were therefore more susceptible to infection. Out of 383 confirmed cases, the team evaluated the aggregation and/or dispersal levels in spatial point patterns based on distance-methods and Ripley's K (1977). They showed that in 63% of cases, residences were located less than 800 m from the index case (the first confirmed case of dengue fever). They also applied a spatio-temporal partition method for identifying cases both close in time (less than 20 days) and in space (within 100 m of places of residence), which resulted in 18 independent clusters. Finally, the order of appearance of these clusters revealed that the disease had spread both in the direction of prevailing winds (which can facilitate the movement of mosquitoes) and along the axes of communication.

According to these two illustrative studies, while nearly 60% of the dengue cases studied presented a high probability of local contamination – thus confirming the usefulness of knowing the patients' place of residence – nearly half of them could not be associated with nearby cases, nor had themselves acted as the source of local contamination. In the absence of data on mobility in retrospective studies, different modeling-based methods have been developed to ascertain the role of mobility in epidemic propagation.

## 1.3. Modeling epidemics and daily mobility

The spread of an epidemic can be modeled as an expansion process in time and space. This process is activated by the circulation of individuals and/or groups who move differently depending on their socio-demographic profile and who transmit a pathogen following different modalities.

Geographic research on epidemics has identified three propagation modes:

– The first mode is based on an ordered sequence of places (**hierarchical diffusion**).

– The second one is based on the proximity between places (diffusion by **spatial contiguity**).

– The third one is based on the relocation possibilities of a phenomenon (**jump diffusion**).

However old, these works have remained largely confined to the disciplinary universe of geography and have not been mobilized by other disciplines studying the spread of epidemics.

### 1.3.1. *Mobility, largely absent from the first mathematical models*

A classical modeling approach in epidemiology assigns different clinical states to a host population and models the transition of individuals from compartment to compartment (Kermack and McKendrick 1927). The first clinical state concerns a fraction of the total population that is susceptible (S) to becoming contaminated. Part of this group may be contaminated and join the infected (I) compartment. After a certain period of time, infected people are cured and may develop (or not) immunity against the pathogen (R, standing for *recovered*). It is usually described in the form of stocks and their transitions: S ⇒ I ⇒ R model, where S + I + R equals the total population.

The SIR model is formalized as three differential equations, which describe the evolution of each of the S, I and R clinical states over time and according to an infection force β and a recovery rate γ:

$$\frac{ds}{dt} = -i\beta SI \qquad [1.1]$$

$$\frac{dI}{dt} = i\beta SI - \gamma I \qquad [1.2]$$

$$\frac{dR}{dt} = \gamma I \qquad [1.3]$$

During each time step, the number of newly infected people is described as the product of the capacity β (or force of infection) of an infected (I) person to transmit a disease to a susceptible (S) person, depending on the number of possible $i$ interactions between the two subgroups, S and I. After a certain period, the infected people eventually recover (R) following recovery rate γ – which is inversely proportional to the infection's duration – and acquire immunity. The choice, number and order of the compartments depend on the epidemic studied. For example, clinical state E (Exposed) could be added, characterizing the period after which the host has been infected, has developed a viral load but is not yet contagious. In that case, we speak of the SEIR (Susceptible–Exposed–Infected–Recovered) model. This class of model describes pathogen transmission among the hosts of the same population, while other models make it possible to introduce inter-species interactions.

Ronald Ross was the first to propose a mathematical transmission model for malaria based on a system with two differential equations taking human hosts and vectors into account (Ross 1911a, 1911b). It primarily revealed that below a threshold value of the mosquito population, the malaria epidemic should disappear. The classic deterministic models used in the context of vector-borne diseases thus take up the bases of the SIR or SEIR models and add new compartments describing the different states of the mosquito, their growth and especially their interactions with humans (Derouich et al. 2003). These differential equation systems are solved mathematically and show great sensitivity to the initial parameters. In the case of a highly contagious disease, a high force of infection will lead to rapid contamination of the whole population, whereas a long period of infection implies that more people are sick at the same time. We should also bear in mind that these approaches only model epidemics at a given place, without taking into account human mobility between territories. Nevertheless, the need to integrate statistics on mobility and migration into these models[5] quickly emerges (Waite 1910). However the difficulty in obtaining mobility data and the limitations of computing power/capacity at the beginning of the 20th century did not make such integration possible. Thus, the work of Ross and McKendrick – the basis for modern mathematical epidemiology – lies on the postulate of a total intermixing of the population, where all individuals are likely to interact, excluding socio-spatial structures and individual mobility behaviors.

### 1.3.2. *The first steps of human mobility in the modeling of epidemics*

While conducting epidemiological research on AIDS, Peter Gould (1993) clearly showed the limitations of these models, which were misdirected,

5. "As emigration and immigration vary considerably in different localities, and in the same locality at different times, their influence on the malaria rate cannot be satisfactorily dealt with except in particular cases where the necessary statistics are available; neither would results in general terms be of much practical use."

partial and based on a series of population dynamic models that acknowledged the temporal dimension but not the spatial one. Since the end of the 1960s, so-called metapopulation models have integrated mobility, primarily as population fluxes between the cities and across the country (Baroyan and Rvachev 1967). In the context of epidemics, these are more or less complex models (SIR, SEIR, etc.) that are able to take into account subgroups with different serological characteristics as well as the commuting of individuals between different geographical areas (Sattenspiel and Dietz 1995; Arino and van den Driessche 2003). In concrete terms, the SIR model is replicated according to the number of cities in the urban system. The population volumes for each city are then used for calibrating each of these sub-models (Figure 1.2).

Interaction rules are integrated into the equations to convey the arrival to/departure from a city towards another city. Inter-city population movements among the infected host compartments are explored in depth. These journeys, processed in the form of mobility flow (or travel probabilities), are generally represented by origin/destination matrices. These metapopulation models, still widely used today, provide powerful simulations at the macroscale because national (motorway flow) and international transport (air flow) are the main modes of propagation of a pathogen at this scale (Sattenspiel and Dietz 1995; Arino 2005). Like any model, they require good estimates of the flow matrices between the different zones, and depend on good quality mobility data (Tizzoni et al. 2014).

Simplified versions, with a smaller number of differential equations, have also been developed to reflect the arrival/departure of populations from a territory. The dengue epidemic that took place in Madeira in 2012 was simulated using air traffic towards the island as a proxy for the importation of the epidemic (Lourenço and Recker 2014). Another study adopted a twofold approach: first, an epidemic was simulated in the area of Karachi (Pakistan) – where dengue fever is endemic. This stage made it possible to estimate the number of infected persons. They then introduced infected people into other areas in the north of the country (where dengue fever is seasonal), matching the likelihood of interactions between different country sub-districts (Wesolowski et al. 2015).

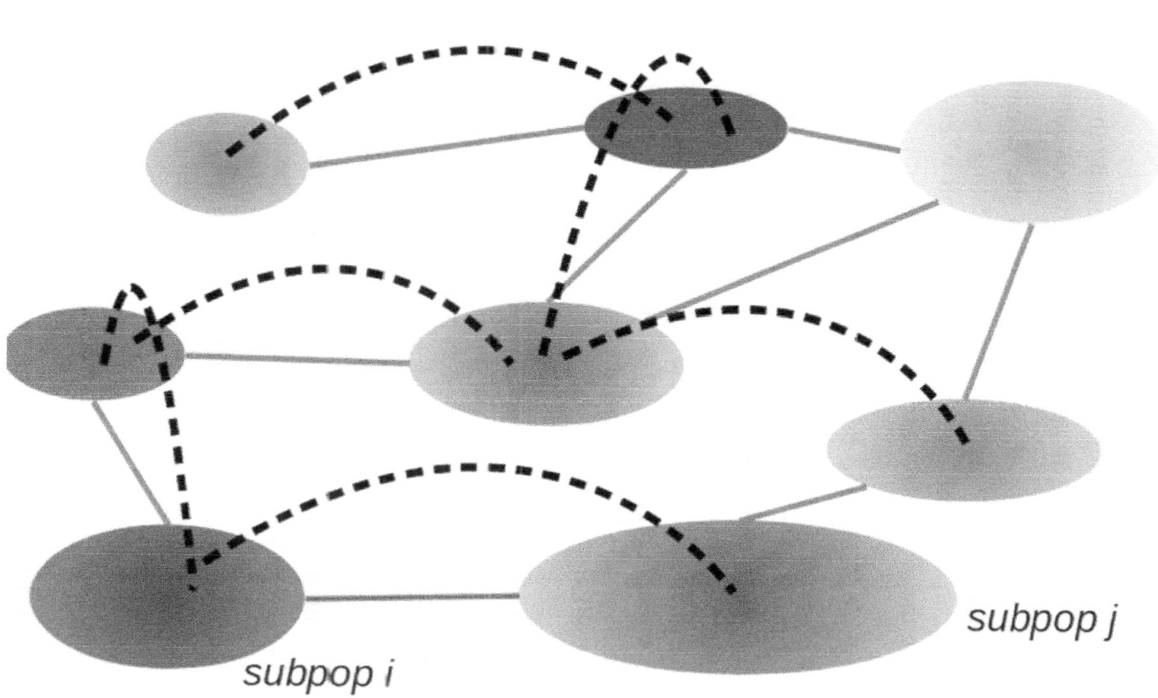


**Figure 1.2.** *Illustration of the principle of spatialized compartmental models, with transport infrastructure (gray links) and inter-city (ellipses) flow (black dotted lines) (inspired by Pastor-Satorras et al. (2015))*

There are solid arguments for choosing differential equation modeling:

– Firstly, it offers the possibility of understanding the global properties of a system through a small number of macroscopic variables (parsimony principle).

– Secondly, all other things being equal, it helps estimate the maximum number of infected persons during an episode if current trends continue.

– Thirdly, it helps to identify threshold effects in the dynamics of a phenomenon. Threshold effects are particularly interesting when several strategies for fighting an epidemic are in competition and when striving to find the path offering the most effect and the fewest constraints.

Yet, these models are hampered by significant barriers to understanding epidemics. First and foremost, the thorough and homogeneous mixing of the population, which results in a lack of consideration for social and spatial structures. This leads to an extremely simplified vision of the characteristics and behaviors of individuals in the population. Even if it is possible to multiply the compartments to represent the different population categories, and to replicate these compartments to signify different territories, calibrating all the parameters that govern these differential equation systems quickly becomes a challenge.

A second limitation of these models: they cannot track isolated individuals and tend to overestimate the propagation phase and epidemic peaks (Ajelli et al. 2010). While these models may be effective in the middle of an epidemic, they struggle to represent and simulate the emergence of epidemics, at the moment when "everything is at stake" by only relying on stochastic interactions between a few localized hosts. They also have difficulty in explaining the forms of diffusion, largely dependent on the spatial structures that existed prior to the epidemic. A necessary complement would require studying the ordinary dynamics of the city and the spaces involving population mobility, alongside inter-host contagion mechanisms, to better understand the geography and local spread of communicable diseases.

### 1.3.3. *Deciphering activity spaces and daily mobilities*

Most individuals travel on a daily basis to fulfill their obligations. They do so regularly (work, education, purchase of goods and services) or occasionally (health, administration). They also travel to fulfill their life plans (socialization, leisure), and all of these journeys are subject to a series of constraints (accessibility, alternative choices in more or less constrained schedules) and opportunities (concentration of activities made possible by urban densification). Depending on the nature of the places frequented, these mobilities can increase or decrease the likelihood of exposure to pathogens.

#### 1.3.3.1. *Complex host–pathogen system*

When stepping foot in different territories, individuals can be exposed to risky environments (Figure 1.1). The pathogenic areas described are in line with the work on pathogen complexes by Sorre (1933). The endemicity of dengue fever in Indian cities is related to environmental conditions (monsoon period, favorable temperatures, availability of breeding sites), letting mosquitoes survive and spread the virus within the population residing within and nearby that pathogenic area. But the environment frequented by individuals is not the only contributing factor to the geography of diseases. Their origin also lies in social factors such as lifestyle or work, individual and collective behavior, resource levels, etc. Disease is thereby considered as the by-product of multiple interacting factors. Through his analysis of the host–pathogen system, Picheral (1983) conceptualized the intertwining of the links between factors provoking, conditioning and predisposing exposure to certain diseases. Health risks are explored as a complex articulation of factors within a complex host–pathogen system.

The concept of *complex pathogenic system* proposes a representation of the global dynamics of an epidemic, pinpointing its elementary entities and interactions. These entities are the pathogens and the prerequisites favoring their development, the possible hosts with their own characteristics and behaviors, and finally, the environmental and societal conditions that evolve over time and are differentiated in space.

The study of a complex pathogenic system is based on the analysis of the different interactions between the system's entities, which act at different scales (or levels), as illustrated by the example of dengue fever (Figure 1.3). Even if a person's vulnerability to a pathogen depends on individual risk factors (age, risky practices, etc.), it also depends on macroscopic context effects (herd immunity, population density). Environmental risk can be measured along different scales, at the level of the district (with the presence of potential mosquito breeding sites) or at the macroscopic level such as meteorological conditions, which influence the vector population dynamics (Daudé et al. 2015).

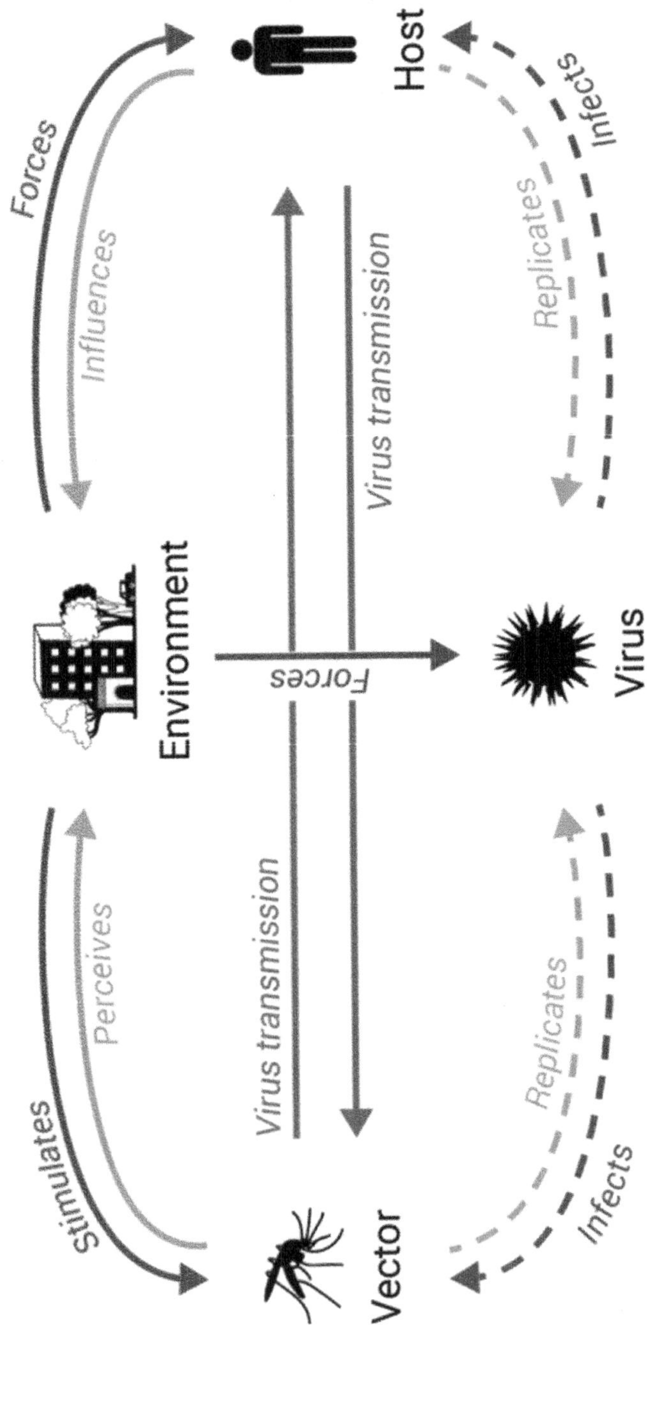


**Figure 1.3.** *Complex host–pathogen system of dengue fever (source: Misslin and Daudé (2017))*

As mobility also occurs at different spatial scales, it can favor the contact between hosts and vectors in high-risk environments. While the mosquito is the viral vector in its living environment (limited to a few hundred meters from its place of emergence, see Ordóñez-Gonzalez et al. (2001)), humans are the main virus carriers over longer distances: at urban (Stoddard et al. 2013), national (Cummings et al. 2004) or worldwide scales (Tatem et al. 2006). The integration of daily mobility then becomes key to understanding the differentiated geography of communicable infectious disease epidemics, in particular at the micro- (neighborhood/district) and the mesoscale (city).

#### 1.3.3.2. *Time-geography and activity space*

The activity space is defined as the portion of the urban space individuals frequent in the course of their daily activities (see Chapter 2). These are all the places frequented by an individual in relation to different activities (work, leisure, etc.). Activities are defined in time (by an ordered sequence of events, as in a schedule) and in space (places in which such activities take place) (Hägerstrand 1970). Depending on their level of spatio-temporal flexibility and the individual's degree of freedom, activities can be classified into two main categories. On the one hand, fixed (or constrained) activities are conducted in predefined places, where individuals do not have much leeway as to their execution time (such as sleeping, working, studying, etc.). On the other hand, flexible activities are less restricted in time and/or space, and require less planning (e.g. impromptu shopping, outings, etc.).

This conceptualization endows each individual with a spatialized time diary, portraying more or less regular events. The study of these activity spaces brings to light the differences between individuals, both in terms of the distances traveled and the number and location of activities carried out throughout the space. They also reveal the spatio-temporal co-presence of individuals in the city. When coupled with socio-economic and demographic information, it is possible to observe mobility and to quantify its potential according to socio-economic status, age, social network size, type of residential area, etc. The differentials in access to basic resources such as education places for the youngest or health systems for the poorest can also be assessed through this approach.

Figure 1.4, inspired by the work of Hägerstrand, shows the activity space for four persons belonging to the same household, performing different activities throughout a day. Each of these activities is associated with different health risks depending on the type of place frequented, the people gathered and the time of day. As the activity space associates an individual with the places frequented, it is well suited to estimate a person's potential exposure to various pathogens (Perchoux et al. 2013). In absolute terms, by cross-referencing all the spatialized time diaries of individuals in a population, and by knowing the incidence rate of a communicable pathogen within that same population, we could calculate the probability of there being one infected person every *n* people present at a place, and therefore predict the contamination risk knowing the number of people present in the same place at the same time (Stoddard et al. 2009; Vallée 2017).

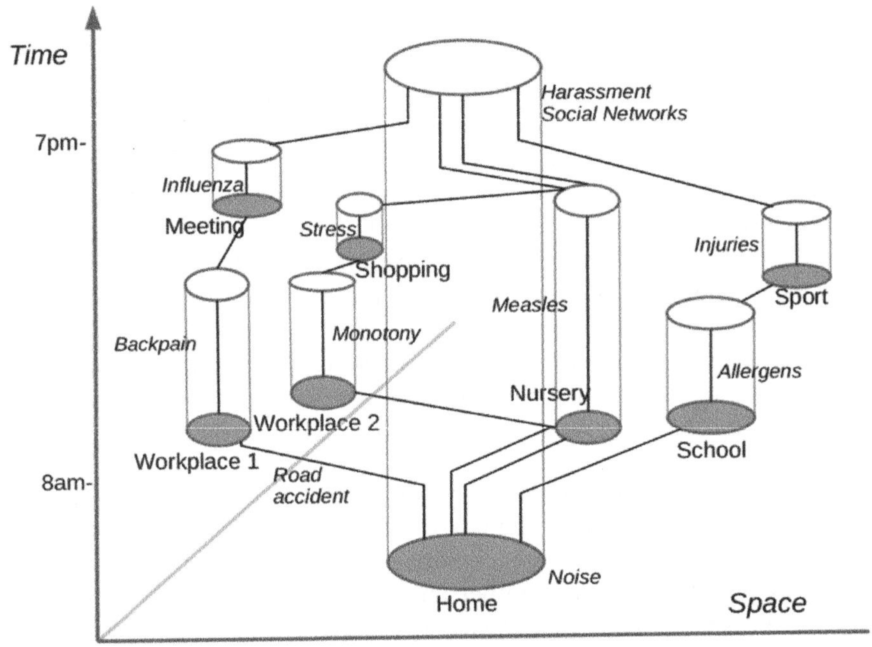


**Figure 1.4.** *Representation of the activity space within a health context (source: Schaerström (1996))*

Taking into account activity spaces and individual daily mobility at differentiated geographical spaces (population density, land use or an ecological niche favorable to the presence of vectors), is the basis for empirical and methodological advances in epidemiology (see Chapter 2) and public health because it feeds the reflection on the production of social inequalities in health (see Chapter 3).

#### 1.3.3.3. *The contribution of agent-based modeling to the study of the role of daily mobility in the spread of communicable diseases*

Together with the theories of complex systems (Morin and Lemoigne 1999) that fuel reflections on complex pathogenic systems, modeling methods have been developed to overcome the obstacles of mathematical models. The challenge is then to model distributed and spatialized processes. In this context, the agent-based model (ABM) has been the main methodological framework used so far (Treuil et al. 2008). These computer models simulate the interactions/behaviors between entities – called agents – in order to better understand the functioning of a system and how it may evolve. Multi-agent systems model and simulate dynamic phenomena in environments in which the individual components are highly heterogeneous, and make it possible to add qualitative and quantitative rules at different hierarchical levels (Daudé 2004; Sanders 2006). These systems can also make it possible to take into account emerging collective structures stemming from the individual behavior of agents. More and more agent-based work in epidemiology is looking into the question of individual mobility, facilitated by the explosion of available data for the calibration and evaluation of these models (see section 1.4). Mobile synthetic populations in a virtual city can simulate activities in various city areas, at different times, following diverse movement rules and tendencies, as well as assess the location/duration of exposure to communicable diseases.

### 1.3.4. *EpiSim: a concrete example of epidemic modeling in urban areas acknowledging daily mobility*

One of the first dynamic models of a communicable disease epidemic represented by an ABM was applied to influenza in six counties in southern California (Eubank et al. 2004). In this model (called "EpiSim"), 18.8 million individuals were generated, living and moving in a space totaling 2.3 million places. These places set up a physical space (home, school, building, etc.), and were connected to one another via a road network graph. Individuals were partitioned into 6.3 million households, whose characteristic distribution was representative of the demographic data of the neighborhoods in the six counties. In addition to belonging to a household, each individual could belong to one or more groups (study group, working group, colleagues, etc.), which facilitated contact opportunities among individuals. In the EpiSim model, each individual had a daily schedule, listing activities with a start and end time, and a venue. These schedules were designed on the basis of a survey conducted on a population sample composed of 60,000 households (National Household Transportation Survey, NHTS). The model made sure that the number of affected individuals in the different locations matched the occupancy statistics for such locations and that the commuting distances from home to work, and between intermediate locations (neither to nor from home), corresponded to those presented by the NHTS.

From this model, different epidemic events were simulated to suit different intervention scenarios: quarantine strategies, vaccination scenarios, mask wearing, avoidance behaviors, school closures, etc. By being modeled at the individual level, the disease and its progression within the population could be followed by tracing the interpersonal contacts at the origin of the contamination and the pathogen's propagation by the individual. In concrete terms, between the moment an individual arrived at a place and left it, the model recorded all of the contact times with other individuals and the subject's relational network dynamic graph. The model was thus able to calculate the disease transmission probability based on the contact time between the infected and the healthy. The likelihood of an individual becoming contaminated during an activity was a function of the cumulative time spent with contaminated individuals. A baseline transmission rate (per contact/hour) defines the risk of transmission.

To go further in inter-individual differentiation, EpiSim models the viral risk of transmission as being equal to the viral transmission rate multiplied by a susceptibility potential and an infection potential. The susceptibility potential, specific to each individual, depends on age, gender and medical history. It is attributed to each agent at the start of the simulation and does not vary. The infection potential, also specific to each individual, depends on the infection stage in the contaminated person, on the treatments administered and evolves throughout the simulation.

Modeling at the individual level, grouped per household, social groups and localizable during the simulation makes it easier to conduct statistical analyses at different spatio-temporal or socio-demographic scales. The distribution per number of daily contacts/per agent is useful to precisely track those who had the most contacts, and thus identify potential "super spreaders". The distribution per contact duration within the population and for each type of activity is used for measuring the dose–response effect and associates it with different types of places or activities. These possibilities offer solutions for many methodological limitations related to the spatial and temporal context in epidemiology. Thanks to them, it is now possible to identify the spatio-temporal co-presences of individuals as well as the contamination contexts of a pathogen that is directly communicable from person to person, or indirectly transmitted via a vector.

For an entirely susceptible population of agents, the introduction of an influenza virus into the EpiSim model offers some lessons regarding the simulation zone. Due to their stochastic character at the early stages of the epidemic, simulation results may vary. This is because the low number of cases at the onset can cause the emergence of the epidemic to fail, slow it down or accelerate it, depending on the location and the first households affected. In a scenario in which an influenza virus is freshly introduced into a totally healthy population, the number of cases at the end of the epidemic reaches approximately 8,650,000 cases, with 46% of the population infected, among which 30% are asymptomatic. Due to the conservation of individual footprints of activities during contamination, the simulations show that the fraction of new infections at home increases from 50% at the onset of the epidemic to nearly 65% by the end of the epidemic. This rises from 10 to 15% for professional activity places, and decreases from 25% to 3% in schools.

Detailed analysis of the attack rate (the number of new cases divided by the size of the susceptible population) also provides accurate information on the progress of the influenza virus. The work of Eubank et al. (2004) showed a strong correlation between the attack rate and the average size of households and the school population share. The attack rate was higher in neighborhoods accommodating large families, where the number of school-attending children is higher. While nearly 60% of the variation in the attack rate by sector was negatively correlated with the per capita income, neither the population density, nor the population per sector were correlated with the attack rate. This last result clearly shows the importance of taking into account individual activities and household composition.

EpiSim illustrates the benefit of an individual-based approach for studying communicable diseases. This approach comprises a variety of risk scenarios, acknowledging the vulnerability of people, population fluxes, responses obtained and timelines. Many scenarios have been tested in EpiSim, providing useful decision-making support for decision-makers: "laissez-faire" to seek herd immunity, opting for an egalitarian or equitable vaccination strategy based on random selection, or for a solution relying on the properties of social networks, for example, by favoring the vaccination of people who have a higher number of contacts than average. As the model is able to generate dynamic networks of contacts by monitoring the agents who are in the same place at the same time, experts can evaluate to what extent the vaccination of one agent, and all of the person's contacts, can be effective at the global level.

Since the first pioneering model, the use of this type of approach has become widespread to other urban areas. But an important obstacle remains: the availability and acquisition of suitable data, in particular, for building activity schedules.

## 1.4. The importance of mobility data in the analysis and propagation modeling of urban epidemics

There are several methods for acquiring daily mobility data, each with its own advantages and disadvantages regarding the collection method or the type of data collected.

### 1.4.1. *Addressing mobility by collecting in situ data, or active data*

Until recently, few solutions were available for analyzing daily mobility. It was necessary to draw on institutional data from a large sample of individuals, data had to take mobility into account, be recent and available in the study area, and a quantitative approach was required. In this context, we are referring to home–work data from censuses or origin–destination surveys (Commenges 2013), or so-called "time use" surveys. For example, household travel surveys[6] in France examine several thousand individuals within the same urban area and provide highly detailed information on the activities performed, the commuting times and the modes of transport used on a certain day of the week. These studies are considered reliable thanks to their proven sampling methodology and contain socio-economic and demographic information. They often serve as the basis for evaluating the quality of other data sets (e.g. Calabrese et al. (2011a); Lenormand et al. (2014)). In the absence of this type of study, or the deliberate choice to carry out a more qualitative or hybrid survey, it is always possible to collect data by conducting individual interviews, either directly or remotely (online or telephone questionnaires).

6. Now called "CEREMA-certified mobility surveys" (EMC²).

For example, Mossong et al. (2008) conducted research by administering a questionnaire to over 7,000 people from eight European Union countries. Not only did they collect information on age groups/gender, but also on the 97,000 persons that the sample members had been in contact with (involving physical contact or not). They also recorded the type of place in which such contact had taken place, as well as its duration. These data were then used to calibrate an epidemic mathematical model used for exploring a variety of scenarios. Thanks to this model, experts can define under which conditions the youngest would be likely to record the highest incidence rates in the case of an emerging disease when the entire population is naïve, and to gauge the effects of specific measures for these age groups.

For the last 20 years, many studies have been based on GPS footprints collected from consenting respondents (see Shen and Stopher (2014) for a literature review or Chapter 2 of this book). For example, based on GPS data elicited from some inhabitants in Iquitos (Peru), Stoddard et al. (2009) were able to reconstruct the activity spaces of individuals, which were then compared to the density of mosquitoes responsible for dengue fever. They then calculated an individual risk level according to the activities performed, mosquito density, and exposure time/duration. In this specific case, places of residence recorded the highest risk levels. After pursuing their study via the contact tracing method (which reflects social ties), researchers concluded that commuting between these places significantly contributed to the local propagation of dengue fever (Stoddard et al. 2013).

When conducted among individuals, these types of GPS-based studies can collect highly accurate geographical information. However, they cannot be applied to too large samples, due to cost reasons (in time and/or labor), nor over too long periods, because they are fairly intrusive and constitute a logistical constraint for the respondent.

### 1.4.2. *Approaching mobility through data collected ex situ, or passive data – digital footprints and online data*

Since the end of the 2000s, technological development in the fields of communications and computing has been characterized by the widespread use of mobile phones and, more recently, social networks. This has been facilitated by improved access to communication networks (better speed, lower prices, technological breakthroughs in mobile phones, etc.). These online and roaming behaviors generate massive data and (sometimes geolocated) digital footprints. As such, they can be used for analyzing individual or collective mobility.

#### 1.4.2.1. *Studying mobility using data from mobile telephony*

A mobile phone that is switched on will continually seek to connect and identify itself with the cell phone tower – base transceiver station (BTS) – offering the best signal (hypothetically the closest one) in order to be reachable or to be able to make a call at any time. The telephone's location can therefore be associated with that of the BTS, which is known. In theory, it is possible to trace a telephone (and its carrier) over time, with a spatial accuracy that depends on the network connectivity of the BTS (Figure 1.5(a)). In France, this spatial accuracy ranges from a few hundred meters in densely populated urban areas to a few kilometers in rural areas. Spatio-temporal information on connections represents a considerable amount of data, not necessarily stored by operators. Furthermore, they are difficult to access for research purposes because operators do not wish to compete with offers they can market themselves. Despite this, other, more "degraded" data can also be accessed. Call detail reports (CDR), which are recorded for practical reasons (invoicing and service continuity) do not offer complete tracking in space/time because the telephone's location can only be tracked when a telephone call (or message) is transmitted or received (Figure 1.5(b)). However, CDR data have the advantage of providing social network analysis based on the number of phone calls between two people. These CDR data have been used for research purposes since the mid-2000s, particularly in the context of human mobility flow studies.

At the urban scale, data from mobile telephony has revealed the high level of spatio-temporal regularity of human mobility, which can be explained by the fact that people spend most of their time in a few places (González et al. 2008). The same team also studied the entropic nature of the mobility of 50,000 users whose regular phone calls sufficed to sow continuous footprints over time. They concluded that 93% of journeys could be predicted, and that this rate was constant in all the population, regardless of the distances typically traveled (Song et al. 2010b). This result should nonetheless be put into perspective. In fact, in cities, individuals often spend most of their time between their home and their workplace, at relatively regular times. There is a high probability that an individual will be present at the same place between two contiguous time periods, especially at night or during working hours. It is also necessary to take into account the level of spatial accuracy, of at least hundreds of meters.

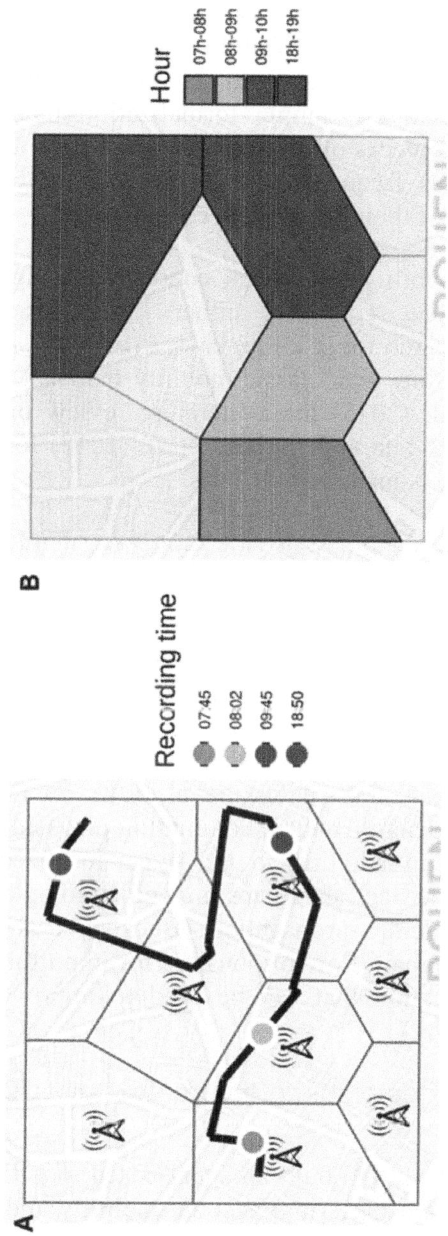


**Figure 1.5.** *Location of a telephone near relay antennas (source: Montjoye et al. (2013)). a) Exact telephone location; b) Voronoï polygons where the phone has been active and where the user will therefore be located according to CDRs*

In line with the work by González et al. (2008), a mobility model has been proposed: the exploration and preferential return (EPR) model. According to this, when one agent decides to change location, they can either visit a new location (with a probability that decreases with the number of locations already visited), or return to an already visited location (Song et al. 2010a). This relatively simple formalization made it possible to reproduce two observed pieces of information at the same time: the increase in the number of places frequented by an individual over time, and the probability distribution of their presence at each place.

Many studies on mobility have been conducted using these telephone data sets in different contexts, either to assess the sample's representativeness, to search for mobility laws, to analyze spatial interactions or to establish comparisons with classic mobility models (gravity, radiative, etc.). See Blondel et al. (2015) for a literature review on the analysis of mobility based on these data and Barbosa et al. (2018) for a more specific review of mobility models inspired by CDRs.

##### 1.4.2.1.1. Telephone footprints in the context of infectious disease outbreaks

A growing number of studies on the relationship between mobility and epidemic propagation relies on telephone footprints. For example, regarding the 2014 Ebola outbreak, Wesolowski et al. (2014) pointed out that rapid and coordinated access to telephone data offered real-time monitoring of epidemic propagation. Data on population dynamics are also essential in the case of malaria at a regional scale (Wesolowski et al. 2012; zu Erbach-Schoenberg et al. 2016), and as for dengue, human commuting plays an important role in epidemic propagation, in addition to the hyper-localized movements of mosquitoes. Despite the fact that gaps in epidemiological data make it difficult to model epidemic propagation (Buckee et al. 2013), they do offer an estimate of the main flow responsible for importing the disease and high-risk areas, information that can be used to improve the monitoring system (Buckee et al. 2017).

##### 1.4.2.1.2. Telephone footprints in the context of epidemics in urban areas

Frias-Martinez et al. (2011) built an agent-based mobility model applied to H1N1 influenza, which takes into account mobility and social networks. Each agent is assigned a probability of being in a cell (a Voronoï polygon corresponding to the spatial influence of the BTS) at a given time *t*, a variable that depends on the day of the week/weekend, all of which is based on location history. The social network aspect is determined by the number of calls between two people, especially when they are around the same BTS, which generally pre-announces an imminent physical encounter (Calabrese et al. 2011b). Frias-Martinez et al. (2011) constrained their model to the following consideration: there was a higher probability of contact between an infected person and a healthy person when the individuals had already contacted each other on the phone and were in the same area. The authors then applied their model to H1N1 cases recorded in 2009 in a city in Mexico. They estimated that the travel restrictions imposed by the government might have reduced the peak of infected people by 10%.

Massaro et al. (2019) studied the influence of mobility on the dynamics of the dengue epidemic in Singapore between 2013 and 2014. To do so, they built daily mobility models, which they then associated with compartmental models describing the interactions between humans and mosquitoes. Drawing on telephone data from 2.3 million people (about one-fourth of the total population), they built an agent-based model reflecting home–work commuting. The place of residence and the main place of activity were associated with the antenna where the person had made or received the most calls or messages at night and during weekdays. They then built three other ABMs (though more related to origin–destination matrices). One of them included places of residence based on CDRs but randomly distributed places of main activity. Another one involved defined primary activity locations in such a way that overall commuting distances followed a truncated Levy distribution, as suggested by González et al. (2008). Finally, in the third model, the places of residence corresponded to those from the census, but workplaces were estimated from a radiation model (Simini et al. 2012). In all cases, individuals move in 320 m$^2$ cells associated with a stochastic compartmental model of dengue. The development of mosquitoes and larvae (larvae mortality, incubation rate, etc.) in each cell of the grid solely depended on temperature. Other parameters, such as the transition rates between E and I, and I and R, were fixed. The number of mosquitoes per human and the number of bites were estimated by calibrating the mobility models in such a way that the correlation coefficients between the simulated and observed dengue cases are closest to the city's scale. Following Lourenço and Recker (2014), they applied a differential equation model for each of the compartments (vectors and hosts), for each cell and each time lapse. In order to be able to follow the serology of each agent, they estimated the new clinical state by performing an independent draw according to a binomial distribution where probability $P$ depended on the total number of people having changed their clinical state in that cell at time *t*. The results of the models were then compared to the dengue cases recorded by the Singaporean monitoring system.

Despite being hindered by some limitations (the entire population is susceptible, only one dengue serotype is taken into account, the infected agents do not change their mobility practices, which are themselves limited to commuting, etc.), the study nonetheless showed that the models inspired by CDRs offer the closest results to observations, both in time and in space, that the diffusion processes of dengue fever in urban areas depend on mobility and are in no way random.

#### 1.4.2.2. *Digital footprints and online data*

The arrival of increasingly sophisticated and Internet-connected telephones goes hand in hand with the emergence of social media platforms. These enable users to interact with the world, and – more or less consciously – to share information about the places visited and the times of such visits: these data are known as geolocated digital footprints. For example, X (formerly Twitter), the popular social network, allows members to share their precise location (GPS coordinates from their phone), by adding content to their message (or tweet). Some social networks have quite large penetration rates at a global scale (e.g. X, Facebook, Instagram, etc.), even if their use varies depending on user age, socio-professional category and geographical area (Facebook is not used in China, whereas Russians prefer Vkontakte).

In the context of research on mobility, geolocated tweets initially made it possible to understand part of the flow at a regional and a global scale (Hawelka et al. 2014; Jurdak et al. 2015). In urban areas, they also showed different mobility potentials matching different social categories in Chicago (Luo et al. 2016) and Delhi (Cebeillac and Rault 2016). By cross-checking these geolocated tweets with land use layers from Google's Points Of Interest (or POIs), individual activity spaces were created, studied and compared with the spatio-temporal discontinuities of dengue fever cases observed in Bangkok (Cebeillac et al. 2017, 2018).

More recently, Data for Good at Meta[7] has provided data on flow that are aggregated every eight hours into relatively large grids covering several kilometers or at a municipal scale, depending on data sets (Galeazzi et al. 2021). These data on the movement of individuals aggregated in time and

7. See: https://dataforgood.facebook.com/.

space revealed the effect of lockdown on local and regional mobility during the Covid-19 pandemic, and favored the study of correlations between the two at these scales (Shepherd et al. 2021). Google and Apple have followed the same path and made aggregated and pre-processed data available, providing information on the activities of users who have activated geolocation[8] on their mobile devices. Nevertheless, as these data are aggregated, they do not make it possible to understand the direct links between individual mobility behavior and pathogen contamination/propagation processes for now.

In line with work that associates areas frequented by individuals and types of activities present in these areas, Chang et al. (2021) have proposed studying the infection places by coupling a SEIR model to geolocated digital footprints. These provide the precise geolocation of nearly 100 million Americans in 10 of the largest cities in the country. They have been offered as part of a cooperation agreement with the company Safegraph, so as to better understand Covid-19. The company collects and cross-references individual and geolocated data with partners and third-party[9] applications, without further information on their origin. Thanks to them, experts can estimate the area of residence as well as the types of places visited (POIs), and the median duration of a visit. Inspired by these data, researchers applied a network SEIR model in which contamination could take place at home or at a POI. The infection rates calibrated by their simulations varied depending on POI size, median visit duration and density of susceptible persons. They were able to show that certain POIs play a more important role in the contamination chain, including restaurants, gyms, bars and cafes – we should nonetheless note that education areas and workplaces were not part of the study. For example, according to their simulations for the city of Chicago, 10% of the POIs represented 85% of the infections. They also detected various vulnerabilities relating to the income level of the area of residence. The mobility of people residing in low-income areas declined less than that of persons living in richer areas, probably because teleworking practices are less widespread or even feasible in the professional categories occupied by the least privileged social classes. Another interesting observation: the types of places that this subgroup frequented were more at risk, with higher population densities, longer exposure durations and higher visit frequencies.

8. See: https://covid19.apple.com/mobility and https://www.google.com/covid19/mobility/.

9. See: https://www.safegraph.com/privacy-policy.

A wide variety of mobility data can be used, either collected directly from respondents or from digital footprints. Their level of representativeness and accuracy (social, spatial, temporal or semantic) conditions their use, both from the point of view of the phenomenon's description and its prospective modeling.

## 1.5. Conclusion

Daily mobility is complex, specific to each individual and variable in time and space. Although it plays a key role in the diffusion process of communicable infectious diseases at all scales, its consideration has only been gradual. First, this can be explained by the complexity of mobility behavior, whose relation to pathogens is difficult to ascertain. On the other hand, the pathogen systems are also complex in themselves. It also took time for the relevant concepts developed in different disciplines to be intersected (geography, computer science, epidemiology, etc.). Technical limitations have to be mentioned, in particular those concerning computing capacities/time, as well as the availability of suitable data.

Although the use of massive data from mobile telephony or geolocated digital footprints is disconnected from their original goal and de facto raises ethical issues in relation to surveillance and privacy, these massive data nonetheless make it possible to better understand daily mobility and to shed light on the diffusion processes of diseases at different scales. Their use in the context of dynamic, distributed and spatialized models is likely to persist over time and undergo significant developments. Among these, a reflection on the association with other databases and the limitations this poses will have to be encouraged. In fact, these telephone data or data from social networks are data without context: no access is granted to socio-demographic information on the profile of individuals, the reasons for traveling, emotional states, the culture of risk or the acceptance of instructions. However, these elements are just as important as mobility when assessing the vulnerability of individuals, and populations, to a certain pathogen.

## 1.6. References

Ajelli, M., Gonçalves, B., Balcan, D., Colizza, V., Hu, H., Ramasco, J.J., Merler, S., Vespignani, A. (2010). Comparing large-scale computational approaches to epidemic modeling: Agent-based versus structured metapopulation models. *BMC Infectious Diseases*, 10(1), 190.

Arino, J. (2005). A multi-species epidemic model with spatial dynamics. *Mathematical Medicine and Biology*, 22(2), 129–142.

Arino, J. and van den Driessche, P. (2003). A multi-city epidemic model. *Mathematical Population Studies*, 10(3), 175–193.

Barbosa, H., Barthelemy, M., Ghoshal, G., James, C.R., Lenormand, M., Louail, T., Menezes, R., Ramasco, J.J., Simini, F., Tomasini, M. (2018). Human mobility: Models and applications. *Physics Reports*, 734, 1–74.

Baroyan, O.V. and Rvachev, L.A. (1967). Deterministic models of epidemics for a territory with a transport network. *Cybernetics*, 3(3), 67–74.

Blondel, V.D., Decuyper, A., Krings, G. (2015). A survey of results on mobile phone datasets analysis. *EPJ Data Science*, 4(1) [Online]. Available at: http://www.epjdatascience.com/content/4/1/10.

Buckee, C.O., Wesolowski, A., Eagle, N.N., Hansen, E., Snow, R.W. (2013). Mobile phones and malaria: Modeling human and parasite travel. *Travel Medicine and Infectious Disease*, 11(1), 15–22.

Buckee, C.O., Tatem, A.J., Metcalf, C.J.E. (2017). Seasonal population movements and the surveillance and control of infectious diseases. *Trends in Parasitology*, 33(1), 10–20.

Calabrese, F., Di Lorenzo, G., Liu, L., Ratti, C. (2011a). Estimating origin-destination flows using mobile phone location data. *IEEE Pervasive Computing*, 10(4), 0036–44.

Calabrese, F., Smoreda, Z., Blondel, V.D., Ratti, C. (2011b). Interplay between telecommunications and face-to-face interactions: A study using mobile phone data. *PLoS ONE*, 6(7), e20814.

Cebeillac, A. and Rault, Y.-M. (2016). Contribution of geotagged Twitter data in the study of a social group's activity space. The case of the upper middle class in Delhi, India. *Netcom. Réseaux, communication et territoires*, 231–248.

Cebeillac, A., Huraux, T., Daudé, É. (2017). Where? When? And how often? What can we learn about daily urban mobilities from Twitter data and google map in Bangkok (Thailand) and what are the perspectives for Dengue studies? *Réseaux, communication et territoires*, 31-3/4, 283–308. doi: 10.4000/netcom.2725.

Cebeillac, A., Daudé, É., Vaguet, A. (2018). Spatial discontinuities, health and mobility. *Revue Internationale de Géomatique*, 28(4), 389–407.

Chang, S., Pierson, E., Koh, P.W., Gerardin, J., Redbird, B., Grusky, D., Leskovec, J. (2021). Mobility network models of COVID-19 explain inequities and inform reopening. *Nature*, 589(7840), 82–87.

Commenges, H. (2013). L'invention de la mobilité quotidienne. Aspects performatifs des instruments de la socio-économie des transports. PhD Thesis, Université Paris-Diderot-Paris VII, Paris [Online]. Available at: https://tel.archives-ouvertes.fr/tel-00923682/.

Cummings, D.A.T., Irizarry, R.A., Huang, N.E., Endy, T.P., Nisalak, A., Ungchusak, K., Burke, D.S. (2004). Travelling waves in the occurrence of dengue haemorrhagic fever in Thailand. *Nature*, 427(6972), 344–347. doi: 10.1038/nature02225.

Daudé, É. (2004). Apports de la simulation multi-agents à l'étude des processus de diffusion. *Cybergeo: European Journal of Geography*. doi: 10.4000/cybergeo.3835.

Daudé, É. and Éliot, E. (2005). Exploration de l'effet des types de mobilités sur la diffusion des épidémies. *Actes du colloque des Septièmes Rencontres ThéoQuant* [Online]. Available at: https://thema.univ-fcomte.fr/theoq/pdf/2005/TQ2005%20ARTICLE%2021.pdf.

Daudé, É., Vaguet, A., Paul, R. (2015). La dengue, maladie complexe. *Natures Sciences Sociétés*, 23(4), 331–342.

Derouich, M., Twizell, E.H., Boutayeb, A. (2003). A model of dengue fever. *BioMedical Engineering* [Online]. Available at: http://dspace.brunel.ac.uk/handle/2438/1692.

Eliot, E., Daudé, E., Bonnet, E. (2012). Interpréter les épidémies du passé : l'exemple de l'épidémie du choléra-morbus en Normandie en 1832. *Geoconfluences* [Online]. Available at: https://halshs.archives-ouvertes.fr/halshs-01082682.

zu Erbach-Schoenberg, E., Alegana, V.A., Sorichetta, A., Linard, C., Lourenço, C., Ruktanonchai, N.W., Graupe, B., Bird, T.J., Pezzulo, C., Wesolowski, A. (2016). Dynamic denominators: The impact of seasonally varying population numbers on disease incidence estimates. *Population Health Metrics*, 14(1) [Online]. Available at: http://pophealthmetrics.biomedcentral.com/articles/10.1186/s12963-016-0106-0.

Eubank, S., Guclu, H., Anil Kumar, V.S., Marathe, M.V., Srinivasan, A., Toroczkai, Z., Wang, N. (2004). Modelling disease outbreaks in realistic urban social networks. *Nature*, 429(6988), 180–184.

Frias-Martinez, E., Williamson, G., Frias-Martinez, V. (2011). An agent-based model of epidemic spread using human mobility and social network information. *Proceedings of the 2011 IEEE Third International Conference on Privacy, Security, Risk and Trust and 2011 IEEE Third International Conference on Social Computing (SocialCom)*, 57–64 [Online]. Available at: http://ieeexplore.ieee.org/abstract/document/6113095/.

Galeazzi, A., Cinelli, M., Bonaccorsi, G., Pierri, F., Schmidt, A.L., Scala, A., Pammolli, F., Quattrociocchi, W. (2021). Human mobility in response to COVID-19 in France, Italy and UK. *Scientific Reports*, 11(13141) [Online]. Available at: https://www.nature.com/articles/s41598-021-92399-2.

González, M.C., Hidalgo, C.A., Barabási, A.-L. (2008). Understanding individual human mobility patterns. *Nature*, 453(7196), 779–782.

Gould, P. (1993). *The Slow Plague: A Geography of the AIDS Pandemic*. Blackwell Publishers, Hoboken.

Hägerstrand, T. (1970). What about people in Regional Science? *Papers of Regional Science Association*, 24, 7–21.

Hawelka, B., Sitko, I., Beinat, E., Sobolevsky, S., Kazakopoulos, P., Ratti, C. (2014). Geo-located Twitter as proxy for global mobility patterns. *Cartography and Geographic Information Science*, 41(3), 260–271.

Jurdak, R., Zhao, K., Liu, J., AbouJaoude, M., Cameron, M., Newth, D. (2015). Understanding human mobility from Twitter. *PLoS ONE*, 10(7), e0131469.

Kermack, W.O. and McKendrick, A.G. (1927). A contribution to the mathematical theory of epidemics. *Proceedings of the Royal Society A: Mathematical, Physical and Engineering Sciences*, 115(772), 700–721.

Langlois, P. and Daudé, É. (2007). Concepts et modélisations de la diffusion géographique. *Cybergeo*, 364, 23 [Online]. Available at: http://193.55.107.45/articles/364res.htm.

Lenormand, M., Picornell, M., Cant-Ros, O.G., Tugores, A., Louail, T., Herranz, R., Barthelemy, M., Frias-Martinez, E., Ramasco, J.J. (2014). Cross-checking different sources of mobility information. *PLoS ONE*, 9(8), e105184.

Lourenço, J. and Recker, M. (2014). The 2012 Madeira dengue outbreak: Epidemiological determinants and future epidemic potential. *PLoS Neglected Tropical Diseases*, 8(8), e3083.

Luo, F., Cao, G., Mulligan, K., Li, X. (2016). Explore spatiotemporal and demographic characteristics of human mobility via Twitter: A case study of Chicago. *Applied Geography*, 70, 11–25.

Massaro, E., Kondor, D., Ratti, C. (2019). Assessing the interplay between human mobility and mosquito borne diseases in urban environments. *Scientific Reports*, 9(1) [Online]. Available at: http://www.nature.com/articles/s41598-019-53127-z.

Misslin, R. and Daudé, É. (2017). An environmental suitability index based on the ecological constraints of Aedes aegypti, vector of dengue and Zika virus. *RIG, International Review of Geomatic*, 27(4), 481–501. doi: 10.3166/rig.2017.00044.

de Montjoye, Y.-A., Hidalgo, C.A., Verleysen, M., Blondel, V.D. (2013). Unique in the crowd: The privacy bounds of human mobility. *Scientific Reports*, 3 [Online]. Available at: http://www.nature.com/articles/srep01376.

Morin, E. and Lemoigne, J.-L. (1999). *L'intelligence de la complexité*. L'Harmattan, Paris.

Mossong, J., Hens, N., Jit, M., Beutels, P., Auranen, K., Mikolajczyk, R., Massari, M., Salmaso, S., Tomba, G.S., Wallinga, J. (2008). Social contacts and mixing patterns relevant to the spread of infectious diseases. *PLoS Medicine*, 5(3), e74.

Ordóñez-Gonzalez, J.G., Mercado-Hernandez, R., Flores-Suarez, A.E., Fernández-Salas, I. (2001). The use of sticky ovitraps to estimate dispersal of *Aedes aegypti* in northeastern Mexico. *Journal of the American Mosquito Control Association*, 17(2), 93–97 [Online]. Available at: http://www.ncbi.nlm.nih.gov/pubmed/11480827.

Pastor-Satorras, R., Castellano, C., Van Mieghem, P., Vespignani, A. (2015). Epidemic processes in complex networks. *Reviews of Modern Physics*, 87(3), 925–979.

Perchoux, C., Chaix, B., Cummins, S., Kestens, Y. (2013). Conceptualization and measurement of environmental exposure in epidemiology: Accounting for activity space related to daily mobility. *Health & Place*, 21, 86–93.

Picheral, H. (1983). Complexes et systèmes pathogènes : approche géographique. De l'épidémiologie à la géographie humaine. *Travaux et documents de géographie tropicale*, 5–22.

Ripley, K. (1977). Modelling spatial patterns. *Journal of the Royal Statistical Society*, 39(2), 172–212.

Ross, R. (1911a). Some quantitatives studies in epidemiology. *Nature*, 87, 466–467.

Ross, R. (1911b). *The Prevention of Malaria*. John Murray, London.

Salje, H., Lessler, J., Endy, T.P., Curriero, F.V., Gibbons, R.V., Nisalak, A., Nimmannitya, S., Kalayanarooj, S., Jarman, R.G., Cummings, D.A. et al. (2012). Revealing the microscale spatial signature of dengue transmission and immunity in an urban population. *Proceedings of the National Academy of Sciences*, 109(24), 9535–9538.

Salje, H., Lessler, J., Maljkovic Berry, I., Melendrez, M.C., Endy, T., Kalayanarooj, S., A-Nuegoonpipat, A., Chanama, S., Sangkijporn, S., Cummings, D.A. et al. (2017). Dengue diversity across spatial and temporal scales: Local structure and the effect of host population size. *Science*, 355(6331), 1302–1306.

Sanders, L. (2006). Les modèles agents en géographie urbaine. In *Modélisation et simulation multi-agents : applications pour les Sciences de l'Homme et de la Société,* Amblard, F. and Phan, D. (eds). Hermes-Lavoisier, Paris.

Sattenspiel, L. and Dietz, K. (1995). A structured epidemic model incorporating geographic mobility among regions. *Mathematical Biosciences*, 128(1/2), 71–91.

Schaerström, A. (1996). Pathogenic paths? A time geographical approach in medical geography. PhD Thesis, Lund University, Lund.

Shen, L. and Stopher, P.R. (2014). Review of GPS travel survey and GPS data-processing methods. *Transport Reviews*, 34(3), 316–334.

Shepherd, H.E.R., Atherden, F.S., Chan, H.M.T., Loveridge, A., Tatem, A.J. (2021). Domestic and international mobility trends in the United Kingdom during the COVID-19 pandemic: An analysis of Facebook data. *International Journal of Health Geographics*, 20, 46. doi: 10.1186/s12942-021-00299-5.

Simini, F., González, M.C., Maritan, A., Barabási, A.-L. (2012). A universal model for mobility and migration patterns. *Nature*, 484(7392), 96–100.

Snow, J. (1855). *On the Mode of Communication of Cholera*, 2nd edition. John Churchill, London [Online]. Available at: http://www.ph.ucla.edu/epi/snow/snowbook.html.

Song, C., Koren, T., Wang, P., Barabási, A.-L. (2010a). Modelling the scaling properties of human mobility. *Nature Physics*, 6(10), 818–823.

Song, C., Qu, Z., Blumm, N., Barabasi, A.-L. (2010b). Limits of predictability in human mobility. *Science*, 327(5968), 1018–1021.

Sorre, M. (1933). Complexes pathogènes et géographie médicale. *Annales de Géographie*, 42(235), 1–18.

Stoddard, S.T., Morrison, A.C., Vazquez-Prokopec, G.M., Paz Soldan, V., Kochel, T.J., Kitron, U., Elder, J.P., Scott, T.W. (2009). The role of human movement in the transmission of vector-borne pathogens. *PLoS Neglected Tropical Diseases*, 3(7), e481.

Stoddard, S.T., Forshey, B.M., Morrison, A.C., Paz-Soldan, V.A., Vazquez-Prokopec, G.M., Astete, H., Reiner, R.C., Jr, Vilcarromero, S., Elder, J.P., Scott, T. W. et al. (2013). House-to-house human movement drives dengue virus transmission. *Proceedings of the National Academy of Sciences*, 110(3), 994–999.

Tatem, A.J., Rogers, D.J., Hay, S.I. (2006). Global transport networks and infectious disease spread. *Advances in Parasitology*, 62, 293–343 [Online]. Available at: http://linkinghub.elsevier.com/retrieve/pii/S0065308X0562009X.

Tizzoni, M., Bajardi, P., Decuyper, A., Kon Kam King, G., Schneider, C.M., Blondel, V., Smoreda, Z., González, M.C., Colizza, V. (2014). On the use of human mobility proxies for modeling epidemics. *PLoS Computational Biology*, 10(7), e1003716.

Treuil, J.-P., Drogoul, A., Zucker, J.-D. (2008). *Modélisation et simulation à base d'agents : exemples commentés, outils informatiques et questions théoriques*. Dunod, Paris.

Vallée, J. (2017). Challenges in targeting areas for public action. Target areas at the right place and at the right time. *Journal of Epidemiology and Community Health*, 71(10), 945–946.

Vazquez-Prokopec, G.M., Kitron, U., Montgomery, B., Horne, P., Ritchie, S.A. (2010). Quantifying the spatial dimension of dengue virus epidemic spread within a tropical urban environment. *PLoS Neglected Tropical Diseases*, 4(12), e920.

Waite, H. (1910). Mosquitoes and malaria. A study of the relation between the number of mosquitoes in a locality and the malaria rate. *Biometrika*, 7(4), 421–436.

Wesolowski, A., Eagle, N., Tatem, A.J., Smith, D.L., Noor, A.M., Snow, R.W., Buckee, C.O. (2012). Quantifying the impact of human mobility on malaria. *Science*, 338, 267–270.

Wesolowski, A., Buckee, C.O., Bengtsson, L., Wetter, E., Lu, X., Tatem, A.J. (2014). Commentary: Containing the Ebola outbreak – The potential and challenge of mobile network data. *PLoS Currents Outbreaks*, 6.

Wesolowski, A., Qureshi, T., Boni, M.F., Sundsøy, P.R., Johansson, M.A., Rasheed, S.B., Engø-Monsen, K., Buckee, C.O. (2015). Impact of human mobility on the emergence of dengue epidemics in Pakistan. *Proceedings of the National Academy of Sciences*, 112(38), 11887–11892.

# 2

# Methodological Challenges of the Cross-Analysis Between Daily Mobility, Environments and Health

**Camille PERCHOUX**
*LISER, Esch-sur-Alzette, Luxembourg*

The study of environmental effects on health dates back to the Hippocratic tradition in medicine (Cummins 2007; Perchoux 2015). Confronted with a severe decrease in the occurrence of infectious diseases and a dramatic increase in chronic ones, it was only after the second half of the 20th century that epidemiology became interested in the contribution of socio-economic, built and natural environments to the promotion and maintenance of health (Susser and Susser 1996). In the 1990s, this line of research became popular as the study of "neighborhood" or "context" effects on health (Diez Roux 2001).

The notion of "neighborhood" refers to "a central living space through which people get access to material and social resources, across which they pass to reach other opportunities, and which symbolizes aspects of the identity of those living there, to themselves and to others" (Meegan and Mitchell 2001, p. 2172).

While it is now recognized that the environments in which individuals live and move influence their health through physical, social, cognitive and psychological mechanisms, the spatial definition of these geographic living environments and the measurement of their attributes are fraught with methodological challenges (Schipperijn et al. 2013; Perchoux 2015).

This chapter references the methodological challenges around the issue of individual daily mobility when assessing environmental effects on health. To begin with, we will introduce the conceptual and methodological importance of taking daily mobility into account when studying context effects on health and, through the concept of activity space (section 2.1). The chapter will then discuss the different tools for collecting data, representations, the characterization and quantification of the activity space in health studies (section 2.2). While taking into account daily mobility offers a fairer appraisal of environmental effects on health (section 2.3), it is accompanied by new challenges in terms of causal inference associated with the selective daily mobility bias (section 2.4).

## 2.1. Acknowledging daily mobility in health studies: the concept of activity space

### 2.1.1. *Limitations of a traditional approach focusing on neighborhoods of residence*

The vast majority of studies on the environmental effects on health have narrowed the spatial extent of geographic living environments to the individual's neighborhood of residence. In the beginning, this was massively delimited at a spatial level and operationalized in health studies by zonings that were predefined, such as administrative residence units (e.g. census areas, postal codes, blocks grouped together for statistical information) (Perchoux 2015). Following the introduction of geographic information systems (GIS) in health studies, zoning with variable size and shape gradually replaced the systematic use of administrative zoning. Circular buffer zones or street networks focusing on the place of residence (Perchoux et al. 2013) became increasingly used. The perceived district of residence has also been the focus of growing interest for delineating the neighborhood of residence thanks to its ability to spatially convey individual preferences, perceptions and experiences of space and its environmental qualities (Coulton et al. 2001; Perchoux 2015; Vallée et al. 2015). However, the main studies on the environmental effects on health focus on the neighborhood of residence: in 2011, over 90% of studies on cardio-metabolic health exclusively considered the neighborhood of residence as the spatial unit of interest for measuring the environmental exposure of individuals (Leal and Chaix 2011).

These "static" definitions of geographic living environments (Perchoux et al. 2013), focusing on the neighborhood of residence, have been severely criticized in many respects. The concepts of "local trap" (Cummins 2007) and "residential trap" (Chaix et al. 2009) call into question the relevance of a local or residential approach for estimating environmental effects on health. Indeed, this approach (whether based on administrative units, buffer zones or perceived neighborhoods of residence) does not take into account the spatio-temporal mobility behavior of individuals and the non-residential environments in which they move throughout their daily activities (Perchoux 2015). Estimating the effects of environmental attributes on health can be de facto biased by the use of zoning techniques that differ from the "real and causally relevant" geographical context individuals are exposed to (Kwan 2012).

This methodological challenge, recently called "The Uncertain Geographic Context Problem" (UGCoP) (Kwan 2012), has two major components:

– spatial uncertainty regarding the identification of the different environments that influence the health of individuals;

– temporal uncertainty as to the individual's exposure duration to such environments.

These two spatio-temporal uncertainties lead to an underestimation of environmental exposures, and contribute to an incomplete – and possibly erroneous – assessment of environmental effects on health.

In this line of thought, "contextual expology" is a sub-discipline of the research field studying "neighborhood effects on health", which aims to reduce these two uncertainties by accurately assessing "the spatio-temporal configuration of environmental exposures" (Chaix et al. 2012), with a special emphasis on daily mobility. In particular, this implies a change of paradigm, no longer reducing the spatial definition of environmental exposures to places (e.g. the place of residence), but focusing on individuals and their movements in time and space (Miller 2007). This is known as a "people-based" approach (Miller 2007).

### 2.1.2. *Daily mobility: an exposure vector to diversified geographical living environments*

"Spatial polygamy" (Matthews and Yang 2013) is built around the simple observation that, in addition to their neighborhood of residence, individuals frequent other places outside of it, such as their workplace, grocery stores, or places devoted to sporting, social or recreational activities. A geo-ethnographic study carried out on 10 families in a district of Boston (USA) showed that individuals only performed 27% of their daily activities in their residential census tract or in adjacent census tracts, and 73% in other parts of the city (Matthews 2011). More specifically, this 73% included a wide spectrum of daily activity types ranging from work, shopping (food-related or not), social and recreational activities, childcare activities and access to services and healthcare.

On a similar note, a study carried out in Paris (France) within a population of adults showed that domestic activities such as food shopping and the use of proximity services are essentially performed within the neighborhood of residence, whereas social and recreational activities such as going to a café or a restaurant, visiting family and friends, are mainly conducted outside the neighborhood of residence (Vallée et al. 2010). Among teenagers aged 15–19 years living in Philadelphia, Pennsylvania (USA) 71% of the time spent outside their home was spent outside their neighborhood of residence (Basta et al. 2010).

Nevertheless, not all populations show homogeneous mobility behaviors. When it comes to age groups, the youngest and oldest populations generally concentrate a larger share of their activities in their neighborhood of residence, thereby reinforcing the influence the residential environment could have on their health. However, even among these less mobile populations, the neighborhood of residence does not correctly delimit the spatial extent of their mobility behavior (Perchoux 2015). A study carried out in four districts in New York showed that the elderly spent 40% of their time outside their residential census tract, mainly for social activities, shopping or doing physical exercise (Cornwell and Cagney 2017). According to a study conducted in Boston (USA), children spend most of their time in their neighborhood of residence (Robinson and Oreskovic 2013). A matching study conducted in Wellington (New Zealand) showed that they left their neighborhood daily to attend school, visit family and friends, or even go to grocery stores (Chambers et al. 2017). Other individual factors such as poverty (McBride et al. 2019) or traumatic events (Friedmann et al. 2020) are correlated with narrower mobility behaviors, though not constrained by the boundaries of the neighborhood of residence.

Since the daily activities of individuals are not limited to their neighborhood of residence, this does not account for all of the geographic environments having an influence on health (Kwan 2012). This chapter develops the methodological issues related to the analysis of mobility as an exposure vector to environments whose social, built and natural characteristics influence health.

### 2.1.3. *Integrating daily mobility in health studies: the concept of activity space*

The concept of "activity space", inherited from the social sciences and from broader notions such as Wolpert's "action space" (Wolpert 1965) or Lewin's "life space" (Lewin 1936), is an individual measure of spatial behavior that describes all interactions between an individual and the environment.

The activity space is defined as "the subset of all locations within which an individual has direct contact as a result of his or her day-to-day activities" (Golledge and Stimson 1997, Chapter 8) in a defined period of time. Spatially, the activity space is characterized by the location of the places of activity and the distance (degree of spatial separation) between them. It is characterized by three sets of places and movements in space:

– the place of residence and the often numerous and short movements made around it, primarily on foot;

– the places visited on a daily or regular basis to work, shop and socialize, and the movements around these places (also often made on foot);

– movements and trips between the places visited, mainly using motorized modes of transport (Golledge and Stimson 1997).

Time-wise, the activity space is defined by the frequency, regularity and duration of visits at a certain place, over a given period.

The concept of activity space was introduced into epidemiology around 2010 (Vallée et al. 2010, 2011; Chaix et al. 2012; Vallée and Chauvin 2012; Perchoux et al. 2013). It marked a significant turning point in the measurement of context effects on health, identifying and measuring the interactions between individuals and their environment in the course of their daily mobility.

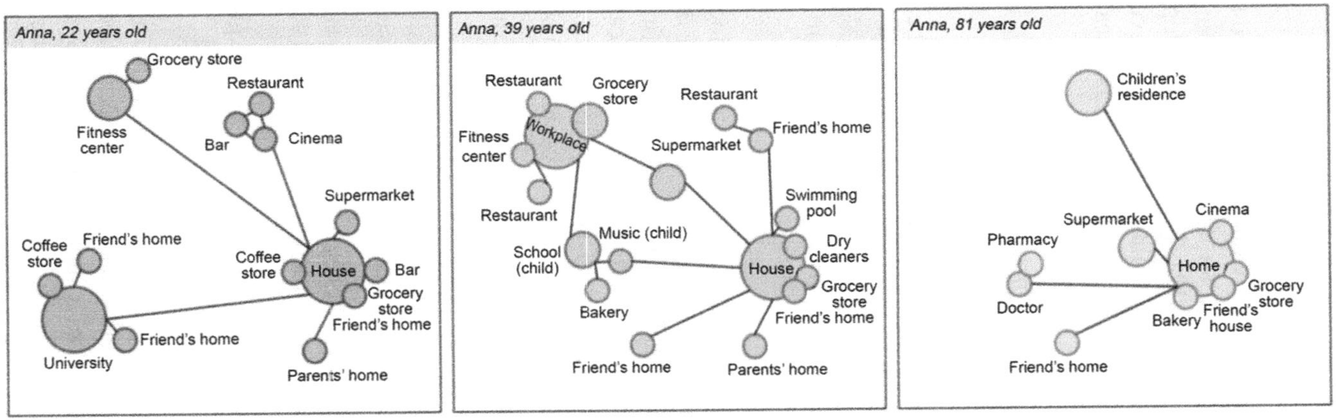


**Figure 2.1.** *Representation of the activity space at different ages (reproduced and adapted from Perchoux et al. (2013)). For a color version of this figure, see www.iste.co.uk/vallee/everyday.zip*

To date, health studies have mainly explored the spatial dimension of the activity space in order to measure the associated residential and non-residential environmental exposures. The consideration of its temporal dimension when it comes to measuring environmental exposure has certainly lagged behind (see section 2.2.3). As shown in Figure 2.1, an individual's activity space is not a concept frozen in time, but can be used to transcribe the evolution of daily mobility over time (Dubreuil et al. 2020). To our knowledge however, there are no longitudinal studies establishing a link between the changes in daily mobility behavior over time and environmental exposures, with a health or health-related outcome.

### 2.1.4. *An interdisciplinary approach to the concept of activity space: understanding individual–environment interactions*

A non-systematic literature review on the assessment of environmental exposure in epidemiology draws on conceptual frameworks derived from time-geography, transport research, environmental psychology and research on social interactions, in order to better understand the structure of activity spaces and the mechanisms underlying the interactions between daily mobility, the environment and health (Perchoux et al. 2013). Based on the results of this study, the three axes presented below offer an interdisciplinary reflection on the concept of activity space applied to epidemiological research.

#### 2.1.4.1. *Defining a hierarchy within the activity space*

Multiple methods for organizing the activity space into a hierarchy have been proposed in the literature (Jakle 1976; Flamn and Kaufmann 2006). For example, the spatial and temporal dimensions of the activity space make it possible to define a hierarchy of places depending on the amount of time spent in each place. In theory, the longer the time spent in a place, the stronger the impact of the characteristics of this place and its surrounding environments on the individual's health. This so-called "dose–response" effect has been observed in the relationship between the duration of exposure to green spaces and stress levels during daily activities (Hunter et al. 2019; Vallée 2021).

Using the concept of a "personal network of usual places", Flamn and Kaufmann (2006) proposed a hierarchy of places of activity according to their relative importance (Flamn and Kaufmann 2006). There are *major* anchor places such as home or workplaces in which individuals spend a significant part of their time and that generally have a symbolic significance; *minor* places of activity that include secondary places of activity such as shops and service places close to the major places of activity, and *circulation corridors* that refer to the routes taken to connect the different places visited (Flamn and Kaufmann 2006; Perchoux et al. 2013).

Finally, other more qualitative approaches could be used for establishing a hierarchy of activity spaces to match the feeling of belonging, the attachment or identity that an individual associates with the different spaces visited, in connection with the activities conducted there and the environmental characteristics of such spaces (Reginster and Edwards 2001; Matthews 2011).

#### 2.1.4.2. *Assessing the constraints associated with the types of daily activities*

Constraints and barriers of multiple kinds (such as physiological needs, physical abilities, environment, distances, time, political, moral, legal, cultural, social constraints, etc.) contribute to shaping our movements and daily activities (Hägerstraand 1970; Golledge and Stimson 1997).

These constraints theoretically have a direct influence on:

– mobility behaviors, shaping individual abilities to move to places or engage in an activity;

– environmental exposures related to the places visited during the aforementioned trips and activities;

– health behaviors such as the use of active or motorized modes of transportation.

The different types of activities (e.g. professional, domestic, sporting, social or recreational, etc.) reflect the constraints on the individual's capacity to engage in a specific activity or trip (Perchoux et al. 2019). For example, shopping for heavy goods, usually done at superstores, involves carrying a considerable load on the way back home. Hence, the physical constraints associated with carrying bulky or heavy goods are one of the major reasons for using a car (Mackett 2003). The type of activity conducted at a certain destination has a direct influence on the probability of getting there on foot (Perchoux et al. 2019). All the more so if the distance between the origin and the destination has an inhibiting effect on the probability of walking; the strength of this inhibitory effect varies depending on the type of activity performed. So-called "discretionary" activities (e.g. free time activities, visiting family and friends, restaurants, bars and cafes), compared to so-called "compulsory" activities (shopping, banking, etc.), would be more flexible in time and space, and more likely to be conducted under ideal conditions such as favorable weather, good physical health, good predisposition or state of mind, etc., thus facilitating the practice of walking and simultaneously reducing the inhibitory effect of distance (Perchoux et al. 2019).

#### 2.1.4.3. *Integrating social relationships into mobility behaviors*

Strictly speaking, social interactions or "social networks" determine the opportunities for traveling, mobility behaviors (Tindall and Wellman 2001) and the distribution of daily activities in space. The distribution of social activities in space, that is, the social activity space, depends on the location of the individuals we socialize with. However, the meaning of places visited for social reasons is different from other places because they do not only respond to the logics of distance, cost or environmental resources, but also to the location of the people we engage with during these social activities (Carrasco et al. 2008a, 2008b). Essentially, social activity places are not interchangeable in the way two supermarkets can be (Carrasco et al. 2008b).

In this sense, the spatial and temporal dimensions of the activity space could be proportional to the geography of social networks (Axhausen 2008). Social networks and social interactions could significantly contribute to defining the number, variety, frequency and duration of visits to places of activity as well as geographic living environments individuals are exposed to (Kestens et al. 2016, 2017; Naud et al. 2020). Briefly stated, the question is not only "where" do individuals travel, but also involves understanding "for whom" or "with whom" do they travel and "why" do they choose to visit certain places or engage in certain activities (Kestens et al. 2017).

## 2.2. Activity space: from the concept to its measurement

### 2.2.1. *Measurement tools and congruence between representations of the activity space*

Since the emergence of the concept of activity space in epidemiology, various data collection tools have been used to quantify mobility. We can mention the use of non-spatialized questionnaires (e.g. the Lawton Instrumental Activities of Daily Living (IADL) Scale) (Letellier et al. 2019) or questionnaires taking space into account, but not permitting the geolocation of daily activities (e.g. Action Space Questionnaire). For example, the Life Space Questionnaire (Stalvey et al. 1999) spans a defined period of time and evaluates how often an individual moves across different hierarchically nested and distant areas from home (e.g. home/garden, nearby residential area, municipality, etc.) (Fillekes et al. 2019a).

Other works have used travel diary surveys and activity logs to geolocate daily activities (Schönfelder and Axhausen 2003). Activity questionnaires combined with interactive mapping make it possible to collect additional information on daily activities (i.e. type of activity, frequency of visit, activity performed alone or accompanied, etc.) while geolocating them on a map (Chaix et al. 2012; Hinrichs et al. 2020). For example, the VERITAS (Visualization and Evaluation of Route Itineraries, Travel Destinations and Activity Spaces) questionnaire developed at the RECORD (Residential Environment and CORonary heart Disease) study in Paris can geolocate 22 types of regularly visited places (Chaix et al. 2012). While activity spaces derived from self-reported activity questionnaires are likely to be affected through memory bias, the advent of GPS has facilitated the collection of objective mobility data at more accurate spatial and temporal scales. While a GPS offers information on individual mobility over a determined and limited period of time, these data are not necessarily representative of the regular daily mobility that is captured by the VERITAS-type questionnaires. Although the majority of GPS studies use seven-day data collection protocols, it is recommended that a minimum of 14 days of valid GPS data be collected to measure activity space (Zenk et al. 2018).

Finally, social media platforms such as X (formerly Twitter) or Facebook have been used for representing individual activity spaces (Lee et al. 2016; Hu et al. 2020), despite the fact that these representations are directly impacted by the limited use of geotags (e.g. less than 1% of tweets are geolocated (Sloan and Morgan 2015)), the low diversity types of geocoded places and the limited representativeness of the population using social networks in comparison with the general population.

Spatial congruence[1] between these different measurement tools was examined and compared to GPS data, generally used as reference measurement. GPS indicators and the Life Space Questionnaires showed a

1. Herein defined as the agreement or superposition in space of different representations of the activity space depending on the methods used to collect individual daily mobility data.

concordance rate of 58% (Fillekes et al. 2019a). Activity logs showed reasonable accuracy, enabling the geolocation of over 77% visits to fast food restaurants and supermarkets via GPS records (Scully et al. 2017). Finally, geolocated activity questionnaires showed relatively high agreement rates with GPS data, although these varied depending on the studies and comparison methods used (Shareck et al. 2013; Kestens et al. 2018; Zenk et al. 2019; Hinrichs et al. 2020).

On average, 73–75% of business locations geolocated through the use of questionnaires are set within a 100–400 m radius from a place of activity recorded with a GPS (Shareck et al. 2013; Zenk et al. 2019). Conversely, a study comparing GPS data to data collected through the VERITAS geolocated daily activities questionnaire showed that over half of the study population spent 86% of GPS tracking time within 500 m of the activity locations geolocated through the questionnaire (Kestens et al. 2018). The high spatial congruence between localized activity questionnaires and GPS data shows that these questionnaires provide valid representations of the places visited regularly, although they are unable to represent the entire spatial extent of individual daily mobility and its variability depending on the type of surveying day (weekday vs. weekend) (Kestens et al. 2018) and the length of the data collection period.

### 2.2.2. *The geometry of activity spaces and health*

These different representations have made it possible to qualify and quantify individual mobility. Different dimensions related to the geometry of the activity space have been identified. These include size (spatial extent), centering on the neighborhood of residence, volume of activities, specialization of activities, the extension of the activity space and its centrality (Perchoux et al. 2014; Fillekes et al. 2019b; Hasanzadeh et al. 2019).

The geometry of the activity space has been examined as a predictor of health behaviors and health conditions. An activity space of a limited size, centered on the neighborhood of residence and displaying a high volume of activity would promote active transport (Harding 2013; Perchoux et al. 2014). An activity space of a limited size, centered on the neighborhood of residence, also limits the frequency of recourse to care, in particular for the inhabitants who live in areas in which the density of doctors is low (Vallée et al. 2010; Vallée and Chauvin 2012). An activity space of a small size could be a protective factor against depression for individuals living in a socio-economically advantaged district; conversely, it would constitute a greater risk factor for depression in individuals residing in disadvantaged districts (Vallée et al. 2011). The size of the activity space is correlated with the perceived health status (Hasanzadeh et al. 2017). However, the size and shape of the activity space showed no association with diet quality, perceived stress, obesity or diabetes (Drewnowski et al. 2019).

### 2.2.3. *Measurement of environmental exposure according to the different representations of the activity space*

Regardless of their geometry, the spatial and temporal representations of activity spaces are used for measuring environmental exposure in relation to daily mobility. The systematic literature review established by Smith et al. (2019) on the use of activity spaces in the study of physical activity provides a detailed overview of this (Smith et al. 2019).

#### 2.2.3.1. *Spatial representations of the activity space*

The most commonly used representations include (Smith et al. 2019):

– buffer zones of varying sizes around the places of activity and GPS tracklogs (Figure 2.2(a) and (d));

– standard deviation ellipses whose orientation and compactness depend on the spatial distribution of places of activity and GPS tracklogs (Figure 2.2(b) and (e));

– convex hulls representing the smallest polygon making it possible to group a set of points (Figure 2.2(c) and (f)).

These spatial representations condition the way in which environmental exposures are measured (Perchoux et al. 2019). For example, buffer zones around visited activity locations or GPS tracks take only visited places into account, whereas convex hulls or standard deviation ellipses include both the visited places and accessible areas, although these may not have necessarily been visited. Different representations of the activity space are likely to produce different results regarding the associations between environment and health (Laatikainen et al. 2018).

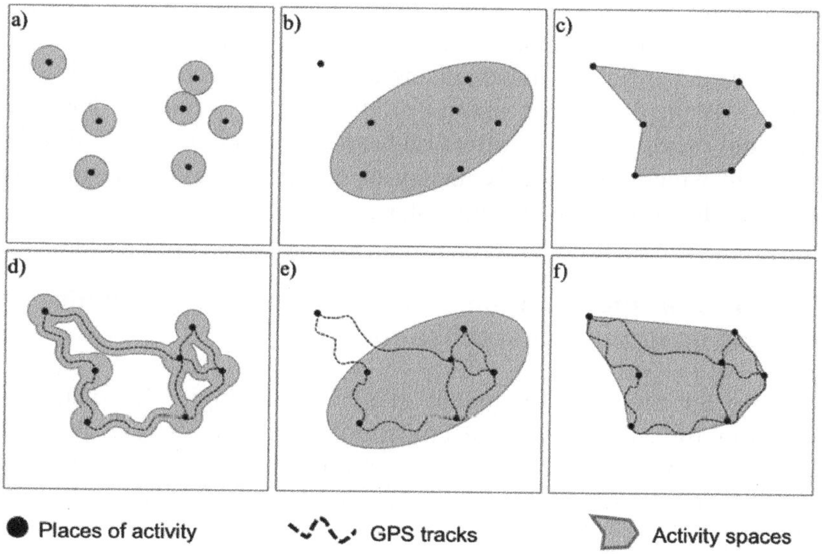


**Figure 2.2.** *Spatial representations of the activity space (reproduced and adapted from Smith et al. (2019)). For a color version of this figure, see www.iste.co.uk/vallee/everyday.zip*

### 2.2.3.2. *Temporal representations of the activity space*

The visit frequency, the duration of exposure to certain places of activity, or travel times, are rarely taken into account in the modeling of the activity space. However, a precise representation of the temporal dimension of the activity space would make it possible to weight environmental exposure depending on the time spent in each location.

Among the simplest models is the use of buffer zones around the places visited, whose size varies depending on visit frequency: larger buffer zones are applied around the more frequently visited places (e.g. residences, workplaces), where individuals are likely to spend a longer time and have more contact with surrounding environments (Perchoux et al. 2015, 2016; Li et al. 2018). Other more complex models take into account the time spent at the place of activity or along the road depending on the traveling speed and the mode of transport to weight environmental exposures (Jankowska et al. 2015; Wang et al. 2018; Scully et al. 2019; Jankowska et al. 2021). Beyond favoring a more individualized measurement of environmental exposure, taking into account the temporal dimension of the activity space questions the environment's influence mechanisms on health (Perchoux et al. 2019). For example, is there a dose–response relationship between the duration of environmental exposure and its effect on health? Can we observe a threshold effect through which a certain frequency or duration of exposure may have an increased effect on health? (Jankowska et al. 2015)

## 2.3. Towards a more precise estimation of the relationship between the environment and health

Thanks to the recent development of new technologies for quantifying individual mobility, the number of epidemiological studies referring to the concept of activity space to measure environmental exposure in relation to daily mobility has increased exponentially over the past decade.

It is interesting to observe that these fields of application are as numerous as they are varied, including the study of health behaviors such as:

– recreational physical activity or transport-related physical activity (Perchoux et al. 2015, 2019; Smith et al. 2019);

– tobacco use (Shareck et al. 2016, 2020; Kowitt and Lipperman-Kreda 2020; Lipperman-Kreda et al. 2020), use of alcohol and other substances (Byrnes et al. 2015; Mason et al. 2015; Freisthler et al. 2019);

– eating behaviors (Zenk et al. 2011; Gustafson et al. 2013; Widener et al. 2018; Drewnowski et al. 2019; Li and Kim 2020; Liu et al. 2020; Raskind et al. 2020);

– access to healthcare (Sherman et al. 2005; Vallée et al. 2010; Traoré et al. 2020).

Numerous studies have also examined how environmental exposures resulting from daily mobility contribute to defining cardio-metabolic health profiles (Kestens et al. 2012; Lebel et al. 2012; Colabianchi et al. 2014; Kimbro et al. 2017; Tamura et al. 2017, 2018; Drewnowski et al. 2019; Raskind et al. 2020; Sharp and Kimbro 2021), mental health (Vallée et al. 2011; Mennis et al. 2018; Zhang et al. 2018; Letellier et al. 2019; Sturge et al. 2020), perceived health (Inagami et al. 2007; Sharp et al. 2015) and some infectious diseases (Worrell et al. 2017).

The sum of these empirical studies constitutes a reservoir of scientific evidence on the contribution of taking daily mobility into account in:

– the measurement of environmental exposure;

– the estimation of environmental effects on health.

### 2.3.1. *Quantification of environmental exposure measurement errors*

Since daily mobility contributes to the characterization of the geographical living environment, limiting the measurement of environmental exposures solely to the neighborhood of residence leads to a biased measurement of environmental exposure. The comparison between environmental exposure measurements in the neighborhood of residence and the activity space quantifies the gap in this measurement error.

The attributes of the residential and non-residential built environment (e.g. utility destinations, transport infrastructure, road traffic) seem significantly different in over 90% of the cases (Hurvitz and Moudon 2012). Foodscapes, in the form of spatial accessibility in supermarkets (Christian 2012; Hurvitz and Moudon 2012), fast food outlets (Kestens et al. 2010) and so-called "healthy" grocery stores (Li and Kim 2020) are strikingly different in the neighborhood of residence and the activity space, showing more pronounced social gradients in the activity space (Kestens et al. 2010; Li and Kim 2020) (see Chapter 3). Environments promoting physical activity and walking are no exception (Tribby et al. 2015; Perchoux et al. 2016). A comparison of "walkability" measures between residential neighborhoods and non-residential activity spaces exhibits similar exposures in terms of urban density in only 21% of cases, 32% in terms of pedestrian access, 35% concerning road safety, 45% in terms of amenities and 46% in terms of crime (Tribby et al. 2015). Finally, exposure to noise and pollution are also subject to measurement errors (Duncan et al. 2017; Ma et al. 2020; Kim and Kwan 2021).

Beyond illustrating the direct influence of the spatial definition of the exposure area on the estimation of environmental exposures, these differences in average exposure to environmental resources between the neighborhood of residence and the non-residential activity space fall under three types of situations (Kim and Kwan 2021):

– Situation 1: the average exposure to these environmental resources is higher in the neighborhood of residence. This means that when an individual travels outside the neighborhood, they visit neighborhoods with lower levels of exposure.

– Situation 2: the average exposure to these environmental resources is lower in the neighborhood of residence, meaning that the individual has access to areas with higher levels of exposure when traveling outside the neighborhood.

– Situation 3: refers to individuals with similar levels of exposure to these environmental resources in their neighborhood of residence and during their travels outside the neighborhood.

According to Kim and Kwan (2021), the first two situations make individual exposure levels converge towards the average when individual mobility outside the neighborhood is taken into account. The use of exposure measurements only focusing on the neighborhood of residence tends to overestimate the statistical significance and size of neighborhood effects on health (Kim and Kwan 2021). This methodological error is related both to the erroneous estimation of individual exposures and to the calculation of the neighborhood effects mean value (Kwan 2018).

### 2.3.2. *Estimation of the relationships between environmental exposures in the activity space and health*

By considering the interactions between people and places at more refined spatial and temporal scales, activity spaces can provide new information on environmental effects on health. For example, taking into account non-residential exposures increases the magnitude of the associations between neighborhood socio-economic level and perceived health, compared to an approach centered on the neighborhood of residence (Inagami et al. 2007). Another example: while smoking among young adults in Montreal is not associated with the presence of tobacco shops near their places of residence, the prevalence of smoking observed among young adults whose places of activity are closer to tobacco shops turned out to be 36–42% higher than among those performing their daily activities further away from points of sale (Shareck et al. 2016). In terms of physical activity, walkability is positively associated with the practice of active transportation, but the magnitude of the associations varies depending on whether the characteristics of the neighborhood of residence or the activity space are considered. Walkability in the activity space showed stronger associations with active transportation than walkability in the neighborhood of residence (Howell et al. 2017). Similar results were observed on the relationship between mixed land use/motorized travel: the part of the variance explained by exposure in the activity space was greater than the one at the neighborhood of residence (Li et al. 2018).

From an analytical perspective, taking into account each of the places in the activity space and the exposure to environmental resources associated with it, does not proportionally increase the share of explained variance in the health variable of interest. A study on recreational walking examined the contribution of environmental conditions in different portions of the activity space according to the types of places visited (workplace, services, recreational destinations and social destinations) (Perchoux et al. 2015). Taking into account the environmental conditions around recreational places in addition to the place of residence increased the prediction of recreational walking, whereas taking into account the environmental conditions around other places visited (e.g. the supermarket, workplaces, etc.) did not improve the model's performance.

In other words, the promotion of an environment conducive to walking, near recreational places (leisure, sports facilities), could lead to a significant increase in recreational walking and have a greater beneficial influence than a walkable environment around other places of activity, such as supermarkets or the workplace (Perchoux et al. 2015). Other studies on the relationships between the foodscape and body mass index (BMI) have shown that taking into account all or certain parts of the non-residential activity space did not systematically improve the performance of the prediction model (Tamura et al. 2018; Dornelles 2019).

## 2.4. The importance of the "selective daily mobility bias" or the impact of individual preferences in daily mobility

Taking daily mobility into account in the measurement of environmental exposure is not necessarily synonymous with a better estimation of causality relationships between the characteristics of geographical environments and health (Chaix et al. 2013; Perchoux et al. 2019). As with the "residential selection bias" (Boone-Heinonen et al. 2011), whose confounding effect results from the impact of unmeasured factors relating to the selection of neighborhoods of residence (see Box 2.1), the studies cross-analyzing the environment, daily mobility and health are likely to be affected by the "selective daily mobility bias" (Chaix et al. 2012, 2013).

The residential mobility bias refers to the selection phenomenon of the place of residence matching individual preferences, which has an impact both on exposure and on the behavior of interest, for example, on health behavior (Diez Roux 2004). In fact, some individuals choose to move into certain neighborhoods precisely with the idea of benefiting from the available resources (e.g. green spaces), with the expectation that they will achieve certain behaviors they attach an interest to, for example the daily practice of running. Taking the example of running, this could result both from the residential exposure to green spaces effect, and from the effect of the interest shown in the practice of running (Boone-Heinonen et al. 2011).

Residential selection can therefore constitute an important source of bias in studies investigating the effect of the characteristics of the neighborhood of residence on health, and a fortiori on health behaviors. To minimize the impact of this bias, different methodological approaches have been developed, and are referenced in the publication by Boone-Heinonen et al. (2011). These methods include the use of longitudinal study designs, statistical adjustment to individual attitudes and preferences, adjustment to observed predictors on residence selection, and the use of instrumental variables. For further details on these different methods, see Boone-Heinonen et al. (2011).

**Box 2.1.** *The residential selection bias*

### 2.4.1. *Selective daily mobility bias: definition*

In terms of causality, one of the major difficulties of studies taking daily mobility into account stems from the fact that the movements observed, the places of activity visited and the associated environmental exposures, are the result of individual decision-making processes based on preferences and values, as well as on environmental characteristics (Perchoux et al. 2019). The "selective daily mobility bias" is derived from the fact that spatial accessibility measures to environmental resources are calculated from places of activity visited with the intention of performing a behavior of interest, and are used as a predictor for this same behavior of interest (Chaix et al. 2012, 2013).

For example, a study on the relationship between spatial accessibility to sports equipment and sports practice could be biased if the levels of accessibility to sports equipment were measured from the sports equipment visited for individual preference reasons rather than spatial accessibility reasons (Shrestha et al. 2019). In this sense, individual preferences (e.g. the desire to practice a certain sport in a certain environment) would themselves be the cause of the visit to the sports facility, while spatial accessibility to sports equipment would not be the cause itself (Shrestha et al. 2019).

### 2.4.2. *The impact of selective daily mobility bias*

In studies examining the environmental impact on health, the selective daily mobility bias could have a more confounding effect than the residential selection bias (Chaix et al. 2013). While preferences in terms of mode of transport, nutrition and physical activity may influence the choice of residential location, these same preferences could have at least as strong an effect on daily decisions to visit certain food stores, to use certain transport infrastructures or even certain sports equipment (Chaix et al. 2013). However, to date and to our knowledge, no study has empirically compared the weight of these two biases. Selective daily mobility bias may also be stronger in studies on health behaviors such as physical activity, modes of transport or food. Indeed, these behaviors call upon more or less conscious decision-making processes influenced by individual preferences and relying on physical urban infrastructures (e.g. grocery stores, public transport stations, fitness centers). Nevertheless, this bias may also be present in studies that analyze more passive environmental exposures, such as noise or pollution (Chaix et al. 2012).

### 2.4.3. *Methods for assessing and quantifying the selective daily mobility bias*

Thus far, the deployment of empirical methods to assess and quantify the weight of selective mobility bias has been quite limited. An exploratory literature review of the selective mobility bias found 14 publications and two doctoral theses in which the bias was discussed, among which only three studies developed empirical methods to assess it (Plue et al. 2020). Another systematic literature review on the concept of activity space to study physical activity came up with nine studies (out of 47) that addressed a potential selective mobility bias, among which only two empirically circumscribed it (Smith et al. 2019).

The proposed methods for circumscribing the selective daily mobility bias have been theorized in the works of Chaix et al. (2012, 2013) and Thierry et al. (2013), and have been referenced by Plue et al. (2020). One of the most widespread approaches involves filtering spatial accessibility measures to environmental resources, by excluding the places of activity specifically visited to carry out a behavior of interest (Perchoux et al. 2015; Li et al. 2018; Scully et al. 2019; Shrestha et al. 2019). Another possibility is to only retain major activity locations (e.g. place of residence, workplaces, etc.) to measure spatial accessibility to environmental resources (Perchoux et al. 2016; Howell et al. 2017).

The use of a so-called "truncated" activity space, in which only the places visited that are not directly related to the exposure of interest are retained, would theoretically reduce the selective daily mobility bias (Perchoux et al. 2016; Howell et al. 2017; Shrestha et al. 2019). A study on the environmental determinants of recreational walking using mobility data collected by means of a mapping questionnaire filtered environmental accessibility measures by excluding the places the participants reported having visited in order to walk their dog, or to practice Nordic walking or brisk walking (Perchoux et al. 2015). Another study on exposure to foodscapes and visits to fast food restaurants used logbooks to identify fast food visits, and manually removed them from GPS data and from subsequent fast food exposure measurements (Scully et al. 2019).

Some studies have compared spatial accessibility to environmental resources in a "truncated" and in an "entire" (i.e. not truncated) activity space, including all the places visited (Perchoux et al. 2016; Li et al. 2018; Shrestha et al. 2019). These studies have consistently shown that measures of spatial accessibility to green spaces and other amenities (Perchoux et al. 2016) as well as to sports equipment (Shrestha et al. 2019) differ between the two activity space models, revealing higher levels of accessibility within the entire activity space. The exposure to environmental resources tends to vary more significantly across social gradients (e.g. household income) within the entire activity space than across the truncated activity space (Perchoux et al. 2016).

Going further in the quantification of the selective daily mobility bias, Shrestha et al. (2019) compared the weight of associations between spatial accessibility to sports equipment depending on a truncated or an entire activity space, and sports practice. The association between spatial accessibility to swimming pools and the probability of swimming is three times higher when measured from the perspective of the entire activity space than from the truncated activity space. Using measures of spatial accessibility calculated from the entire activity space could lead to an acutely different estimate of the strength of the association between environmental resources and health behaviors. While more studies are needed to conclude on the magnitude of the selective mobility bias, we could observe an overestimation of the effects of the environment on health behaviors of interest, as with the residential mobility bias. The correction of spatial accessibility measures through the use of a truncated activity space may constitute an effective strategy to harness the selective daily mobility bias (Shrestha et al. 2019).

Another method for limiting the selective daily mobility bias, based exclusively on the use of GPS data, involves excluding the GPS tracks corresponding to the paths taken between the places visited, in order to measure the environmental exposures along the shortest path between two places (Burgoine et al. 2015; Chaix et al. 2016; Klein et al. 2021).

The underlying hypothesis is that the environmental characteristics observed with GPS tracks differ from the characteristics measured through the shortest paths, thus reflecting individual preferences in terms of environments and the adequacy between an environment and a behavior or a state of health.

Burgoine et al. (2015) assessed the impact of using GPS tracks rather than the shortest routes from home to school in children aged 5–11 years, for estimating associations between environment and BMI. However, no association between environment and BMI was observed, neither on GPS tracks nor with the shortest path method. Therefore, no identification of a potential selective daily mobility bias could be established in this study.

Another study by Klein et al. (2021) also compared the environmental characteristics of the paths observed through GPS tracks and the shortest paths according to the modes of transport used (motorized vs. walking), for a population of adults residing in Luxembourg. The results showed a significant difference in exposure to areas with low traffic speeds (e.g. 30 km/h) and street network connectivity between the shortest paths and the paths observed with the different modes of transport, thus revealing the presence of a selective mobility bias. In addition, a greater presence of service facilities, street network connectivity, green spaces and areas with low traffic speeds was associated with an increase in the percentage of detours between the observed paths and the shortest paths for journeys made on foot (Klein et al. 2021).

The discrepancies in the results by Burgoine et al. on the one hand, and the above-mentioned studies by Shrestha et al. and Klein et al. on the other hand, could be attributable to the fact that the "causal chain" linking accessibility to environmental resources along the paths taken and BMI is more distal than the one linking spatial accessibility to sports equipment and the practice of sports activities, or the one associating the environmental characteristics of the paths taken with the modes of transport used (Shrestha et al. 2019; Klein et al. 2021).

Finally, a last, more complex method should evaluate whether the behavior of interest, observed at a given place and time, results from the environmental opportunities observed at the places visited just before or just after said behavior (Thierry et al. 2013; Chaix et al. 2016). A study on the relationship between the built environment and walking, relying on GPS data and considering the probability of walking as the unit of analysis, attempted to reduce the selective mobility bias by taking into account the modes of transport used during the previous trip (Chaix et al. 2016). Not only did the mode of transport of the previous trip influence the environmental characteristics of the place visited (e.g. a pedestrian preferably moved towards a destination whose environment was favorable to walking), but also the mode of transport of the subsequent journey (e.g. the same mode of transport was often used for the round trip) (Chaix et al. 2016).

### 2.4.4. *Selective daily mobility bias: what generalization?*

The theoretical importance of the selective daily mobility bias makes it essential to identify and quantify it in studies taking individual mobility into account to assess environmental effects on health behaviors. However, the small number of studies that have empirically assessed the presence (or absence) of this bias does not currently allow us to generalize the results observed in terms of the bias strength (Plue et al. 2020).

The heterogeneity of methods used for calculating accessibility to environmental resources and to filter these exposures according to selection processes related to individual preferences contributes to reducing the comparability between studies. In addition, some methods, such as the use of truncated activity spaces, have been discussed in view of their overly drastic exposure filtering approach, which could lead to both removing the source of the bias and losing contextual information to explain the individual choice and behavior logic (Li et al. 2018; Plue et al. 2020), in particular when it comes to accumulating environmental exposure.

Despite their complexity, a call has been made for more flexible methods that can simultaneously take into account the places visited and the routes taken (Plue et al. 2020). Finally, the methods used to take this bias into account can be ambitious in terms of the data to be collected, and require multiple collection tools (e.g. logbooks, activity logs, interviews, Ecological Momentary Assessment questionnaires). While GPS data allow us to answer questions such as "where or when" (Kestens et al. 2017) individuals interact with their geographic living environments, they provide little contextual information on the type of activity performed, the "what" (Perchoux et al. 2019) and decision-making processes, the "why" (Plue et al. 2020), including selection phenomena, which lead to adopting a specific behavior at a given place and time.

## 2.5. Conclusion: towards new methodological developments

The cross-analysis of geographical environments and health generates many methodological challenges pertaining to the integration of daily mobility. By exploring these challenges in depth, this chapter has stressed that the estimation of associations between environment and health, as well as the causal interpretation of results, are closely related to the definition and operationalization of daily mobilities and the geographical environments derived from them.

In addition to the aforementioned methodological challenges, new so-called "ecological" approaches make it possible to collect additional information on environment–individual interactions, synchronously in time and space. More specifically, the Ecological Momentary Assessment (EMA), often issued by means of a questionnaire on a smartphone, repeatedly collects information about the participant's behavior, attitude, experience, environment, all in real time.

Coupled with GPS data, EMAs are becoming explicit "Geographic Momentary Ecological Assessment" sheets (GEMAs), capturing the locations of individuals during their responses to EMAs and linking them to objective environmental data via geographic information systems.

GEMAs have been used in particular to collect momentary data on the perceived environment, subjective experiences (such as emotions, stress) or even health behaviors. The outpatient assessment of individual subjective experience can also be supplemented with various sensors so as to passively and objectively collect environmental observations (e.g. air pollution, noise pollution, social interactions via Wi-Fi), behavioral indicators (e.g. accelerometer) or physiological markers (such as electrodermal activity, heart rate, skin temperature, glucose, etc.).

More interventional study designs have capitalized on recent developments in terms of virtual reality or augmented reality to examine environment–mobility–health interactions. Often taking the form of stated preference experiments, a small but growing number of researchers have used immersive virtual environments combined with walking or biking simulators to examine environmental preferences and emotions associated with mobility behaviors in controlled environments (Bialkova et al. 2018; Birenboim et al. 2019, 2021; Lieze et al. 2020). The potential of virtual reality to reproduce complex and highly realistic built environments while controlling *stimuli* and external confounding factors (e.g. sound environment) provides a high internal validity to these studies (Birenboim et al. 2021).

While this chapter has tried to expose the methodological challenges related to the cross-analysis of mobility and health, it is important to note that these methods have opened up new opportunities to better understand the interactions between individuals and their geographical environments, at refined spatial and temporal scales.

## 2.6. References

Axhausen, K.W. (2008). Social networks, mobility biographies, and travel: Survey challenges. *Environment and Planning B: Planning and Design*, 35(6), 981–996. doi: 10.1068/b3316t.

Basta, L.A., Richmond, T.S., Wiebe, D.J. (2010). Neighborhoods, daily activities, and measuring health risks experienced in urban environments. *Social Science and Medicine*, 71(11). doi: 10.1016/j.socscimed.2010.09.008.

Bialkova, S., Ettema, D., Dijst, M. (2018). Urban future: Unlocking cycling with VR applications. *2018 IEEE Workshop on Augmented and Virtual Realities for Good, VAR4Good 2018*. doi: 10.1109/VAR4GOOD. 2018.8576888.

Birenboim, A., Dijst, M., Ettema, D., de Kruijf, J., de Leeuw, G., Dogterom, N. (2019). The utilization of immersive virtual environments for the investigation of environmental preferences. *Landscape and Urban Planning*, 189. doi: 10.1016/j.landurbplan.2019.04.011.

Birenboim, A., Ben-Nun Bloom, P., Levit, H., Omer, I. (2021). The study of walking, walkability and wellbeing in immersive virtual environments. *International Journal of Environmental Research and Public Health*, 18(2), 364.

Boone-Heinonen, J., Gordon-Larsen, P., Guilkey, D.K., Jacobs Jr, D.R., Popkin, B.M. (2011). Environment and physical activity dynamics: The role of residential self-selection. *Psychology of Sport and Exercise*, 12(1), 54–60.

Burgoine, T., Jones, A.P., Namenek Brouwer, R.J., Benjamin Neelon, S.E. (2015). Associations between BMI and home, school and route environmental exposures estimated using GPS and GIS: Do we see evidence of selective daily mobility bias in children? *International Journal of Health Geographics*, 14(1). doi: 10.1186/1476-072X-14-8.

Byrnes, H.F., Miller, B.A., Wiebe, D.J., Morrison, C.N., Remer, L.G., Wiehe, S.E. (2015). Tracking adolescents with global positioning system-enabled cell phones to study contextual exposures and alcohol and marijuana use: A pilot study. *Journal of Adolescent Health*, 57(2). doi: 10.1016/j.jadohealth.2015.04.013.

Carrasco, J.A., Hogan, B., Wellman, B., Miller, E.J. (2008a). Agency in social activity interactions: The role of social networks in time and space. *Tijdschrift voor Economische en Sociale Geografie*, 99(5), 562–583. doi: 10.1111/j.1467-9663.2008.00492.x.

Carrasco, J.A., Hogan, B., Wellman, B., Miller, E.J. (2008b). Collecting social network data to study social activity-travel behavior: An egocentric approach. *Environment and Planning B: Planning and Design*, 35(6), 961–980. doi: 10.1068/b3317t.

Chaix, B., Merlo, J., Evans, D., Leal, C., Havard, S. (2009). Neighbourhoods in eco-epidemiologic research: Delimiting personal exposure areas. A response to Riva, Gauvin, Apparicio and Brodeur. *Social Science and Medicine* 69, 9. doi: 10.1016/j.socscimed.2009.07.018.

Chaix, B., Kestens, Y., Perchoux, C., Karusisi, N., Merlo, J., Labadi, K. (2012). An interactive mapping tool to assess individual mobility patterns in neighborhood studies. *American Journal of Preventive Medicine*, 43(4), 440–450. doi: 10.1016/j.amepre.2012.06.026.

Chaix, B., Méline, J., Duncan, S., Merrien, C., Karusisi, N., Perchoux, C., Lewin, A., Labadi, K., Kestens, Y. (2013). GPS tracking in neighborhood and health studies: A step forward for environmental exposure assessment, a step backward for causal inference? *Health and Place*, 21, 46–51. doi: 10.1016/j.healthplace.2013.01.003.

Chaix, B., Kestens, Y., Duncan, D.T., Brondeel, R., Méline, J., El Aarbaoui, T., Pannier, B., Merlo, J. (2016). A GPS-based methodology to analyze environment-health associations at the trip level: Case-crossover analyses of built environments and walking. *American Journal of Epidemiology*, 184(8), 579–589. doi: 10.1093/aje/kww071.

Chambers, T., Pearson, A.L., Kawachi, I., Rzotkiewicz, Z., Stanley, J., Smith, M., Barr, M., Ni Mhurchu, C., Signal, L. (2017). Kids in space: Measuring children's residential neighborhoods and other destinations using activity space GPS and wearable camera data. *Social Science and Medicine*, 193. doi: 10.1016/j.socscimed.2017.09.046.

Christian, W.J. (2012). Using geospatial technologies to explore activity-based retail food environments. *Spatial and Spatiotemporal Epidemiology*, 3(4). doi: 10.1016/j.sste.2012.09.001.

Colabianchi, N., Coulton, C.J., Hibbert, J.D., McClure, S.M., Ievers-Landis, C.E., Davis, E.M. (2014). Adolescent self-defined neighborhoods and activity spaces: Spatial overlap and relations to physical activity and obesity. *Health and Place*, 27. doi: 10.1016/j.healthplace.2014.01.004.

Cornwell, E.Y. and Cagney, K.A. (2017). Aging in activity space: Results from smart-phone-based GPS-tracking of urban seniors. *Journals of Gerontology – Series B Psychological Sciences and Social Sciences*, 72(5). doi: 10.1093/geronb/gbx063.

Coulton, C.J., Korbin, J., Chan, T., Su, M. (2001). Mapping residents' perceptions of neighborhood boundaries: A methodological note. *American Journal of Community Psychology*, 29(2). doi: 10.1023/A:1010303419034.

Cummins, S. (2007). Commentary: Investigating neighbourhood effects on health – Avoiding the "local trap". *International Journal of Epidemiology*. doi: 10.1093/ije/dym033.

Diez Roux, A.V. (2001). Investigating neighborhood and area effects on health. *American Journal of Public Health*, 91(11), 1783–1789. doi: 10.2105/AJPH.91.11.1783.

Diez Roux, A.V. (2004). Estimating neighborhood health effects: The challenges of causal inference in a complex world. *Social Science and Medicine*. doi: 10.1016/S0277-9536 (03)00414-3.

Dornelles, A. (2019). Impact of multiple food environments on body mass index. *PLoS ONE*, 14(8). doi: 10.1371/journal.pone.0219365.

Drewnowski, A., Aggarwal, A., Rose, C.M., Gupta, S., Delaney, J.A., Hurvitz, P.M. (2019). Activity space metrics not associated with sociodemographic variables, diet or health outcomes in the Seattle Obesity Study II. *Spatial and Spatiotemporal Epidemiology*, 30. doi: 10.1016/j.sste.2019.100289.

Dubreuil, A., Vallée, J., Shareck, M., Frohlich, K.L. (2020). L'évolution des espaces d'activité lors de la transition vers l'âge adulte (Montréal, Canada). *Revue Jeunes et Société*, 5(1). doi: 10.7202/1070526ar.

Duncan, D.T., Tamura, K., Regan, S.D., Athens, J., Elbel, B., Meline, J., Al-Ajlouni, Y.A., Chaix, B. (2017). Quantifying spatial misclassification in exposure to noise complaints among low-income housing residents across New York City neighborhoods: A Global Positioning System (GPS) study. *Annals of Epidemiology*, 27(1). doi: 10.1016/j.annepidem.2016.09.017.

Fillekes, M.P., Röcke, C., Katana, M., Weibel, R. (2019a). Self-reported versus GPS-derived indicators of daily mobility in a sample of healthy older adults. *Social Science and Medicine*, 220. doi: 10.1016/j.socscimed.2018.11.010.

Fillekes, M.P., Giannouli, E., Kim, E.K., Zijlstra, W., Weibel, R. (2019b). Towards a comprehensive set of GPS-based indicators reflecting the multidimensional nature of daily mobility for applications in health and aging research. *International Journal of Health Geographics*, 18(1). doi: 10.1186/s12942-019-0181-0.

Flamn, M.F. and Kaufmann, V. (2006). The concept of personal network of usual places as a tool for analysing human activity spaces: A quantitative exploration. *Conference Paper STRC*. doi: 10.1108/02580540410567256.

Freisthler, B., Kepple, N.J., Wolf, J.P., Carson, L. (2019). Activity spaces: Assessing differences in alcohol exposures and alcohol use for parents. *GeoJournal*. doi: 10.1007/s10708-019-10059-5.

Friedmann, F., Santangelo, P., Ebner-Priemer, U., Hill, H., Neubauer, A.B., Rausch, S., Steil, R., Müller-Engelmann, M., Kleindienst, N., Bohus, M. (2020). Life within a limited radius: Investigating activity space in women with a history of child abuse using global positioning system tracking. *PLoS ONE*, 15(5). doi: 10.1371/journal.pone.0232666.

Golledge, R.D. and Stimson, R.J. (1997). *Spatial Behavior: A Geographic Perspective*. Guilford Press, New York.

Gustafson, A., Christian, J.W., Lewis, S., Moore, K., Jilcott, S. (2013). Food venue choice, consumer food environment, but not food venue availability within daily travel patterns are associated with dietary intake among adults, Lexington Kentucky 2011. *Nutrition Journal*, 12(1). doi: 10.1186/1475-2891-12-17.

Hägerstraand, T. (1970). What about people in Regional Science? *Papers in Regional Science*, 24(1), 7–24. doi: 10.1111/j.1435-5597.1970.tb01464.x.

Harding, C. (2013). Activity space geometry and its effect on mode choice. *Proceedings of the 92nd Annual Meeting of the Transportation Research Board*, Washington D.C.

Hasanzadeh, K., Broberg, A., Kyttä, M. (2017). Where is my neighborhood? A dynamic individual-based definition of home ranges and implementation of multiple evaluation criteria. *Applied Geography*, 84. doi: 10.1016/j.apgeog.2017.04.006.

Hasanzadeh, K., Czepkiewicz, M., Heinonen, J., Kyttä, M., Ala-Mantila, S., Ottelin, J. (2019). Beyond geometries of activity spaces: A holistic study of daily travel patterns, individual characteristics, and perceived wellbeing in Helsinki metropolitan area. *Journal of Transport and Land Use*. doi: 10.5198/jtlu.2019.1148.

Hinrichs, T., Zanda, A., Fillekes, M.P., Bereuter, P., Portegijs, E., Rantanen, T., Schmidt-Trucksäss, A., Zeller, A.W., Weibel, R. (2020). Map-based assessment of older adults' life space: Validity and reliability. *European Review of Aging and Physical Activity*, 17(1). doi: 10.1186/s11556-020-00253-7.

Howell, N.A., Farber, S., Widener, M.J., Booth, G.L. (2017). Residential or activity space walkability: What drives transportation physical activity? *Journal of Transport and Health*. doi: 10.1016/j.jth.2017.08.011.

Hu, L., Li, Z., Ye, X. (2020). Delineating and modeling activity space using geotagged social media data. *Cartography and Geographic Information Science*, 47(3). doi: 10.1080/15230406.2019.1705187.

Hunter, M.C.R., Gillespie, B.W., Chen, S.Y.P. (2019). Urban nature experiences reduce stress in the context of daily life based on salivary biomarkers. *Frontiers in Psychology*, 10. doi: 10.3389/fpsyg.2019.00722.

Hurvitz, P.M. and Moudon, A.V. (2012). Home versus nonhome neighborhood: Quantifying differences in exposure to the built environment. *American Journal of Preventive Medicine*. doi: 10.1016/j.amepre.2011.11.015.

Inagami, S., Cohen, D.A., Finch, B.K. (2007). Nonresidential neighborhood exposures suppress neighborhood effects on self-rated health. *Social Science and Medicine*, 65(8). doi: 10.1016/j.socscimed.2007.05.051.

Jakle, J.A. (1976). *Human Spatial Behavior: A Social Geography*. Duxbury Press, North Scituate.

Jankowska, M.M., Schipperijn, J., Kerr, J. (2015). A framework for using GPS data in physical activity and sedentary behavior studies. *Exercise and Sport Sciences Reviews*. doi: 10.1249/JES.0000000000000035.

Jankowska, M.M., Yang, J.A., Luo, N., Spoon, C., Benmarhnia, T. (2021). Accounting for space, time, and behavior using GPS derived dynamic measures of environmental exposure. *Health and Place*. doi: 10.1016/j.healthplace.2021.102706.

Kestens, Y., Lebel, A., Daniel, M., Thériault, M., Pampalon, R. (2010). Using experienced activity spaces to measure foodscape exposure. *Health and Place*, 16(6), 1094–1103. doi: 10.1016/j.healthplace.2010.06.016.

Kestens, Y., Lebel, A., Chaix, B., Clary, C., Daniel, M., Pampalon, R., Theriault, M., Subramanian, S.V. (2012). Association between activity space exposure to food establishments and individual risk of overweight. *PLoS ONE*, 7(8). doi: 10.1371/journal.pone.0041418.

Kestens, Y., Chaix, B., Gerber, P., Desprès, M., Gauvin, L., Klein, O., Klein, S., Köppen, B., Lord, S., Naud, A. (2016). Understanding the role of contrasting urban contexts in healthy aging: An international cohort study using wearable sensor devices (the CURHA study protocol). *BMC Geriatrics*, 16(1), 96. doi: 10.1186/s12877-016-0273-7.

Kestens, Y., Wasfi, R., Naud, A., Chaix, B. (2017). Contextualizing context: Reconciling environmental exposures, social networks, and location preferences in health research. *Current Environmental Health Reports*, 4(1), 51–60. doi: 10.1007/s40572-017-0121-8.

Kestens, Y., Thierry, B., Shareck, M., Steinmetz-Wood, M., Chaix, B. (2018). Integrating activity spaces in health research: Comparing the VERITAS activity space questionnaire with 7-day GPS tracking and prompted recall. *Spatial and Spatiotemporal Epidemiology*, 25, 1–9. doi: 10.1016/j.sste.2017.12.003.

Kim, J. and Kwan, M.P. (2021). How neighborhood effect averaging might affect assessment of individual exposures to air pollution: A study of ozone exposures in Los Angeles. *Annals of the American Association of Geographers*, 111(1). doi: 10.1080/24694452.2020.1756208.

Kimbro, R.T., Sharp, G., Denney, J.T. (2017). Home and away: Area socioeconomic disadvantage and obesity risk. *Health and Place*, 44. doi: 10.1016/j.healthplace.2017.02.001.

Klein, S., Brondeel, R., Chaix, B., Klein, O., Thierry, B., Kestens, Y., Gerber, P., Perchoux, C. (2021). What triggers selective daily mobility among older adults? A study comparing trip and environmental characteristics between observed path and shortest path. *Health & Place*, 102730. doi: 10.1016/j.healthplace.2021.102730.

Kowitt, S.D. and Lipperman-Kreda, S. (2020). How is exposure to tobacco outlets within activity spaces associated with daily tobacco use among youth? A mediation analysis. *Nicotine and Tobacco Research*, 22(6). doi: 10.1093/ntr/ntz088.

Kwan, M.P. (2012). The uncertain geographic context problem. *Annals of the Association of American Geographers*, 102(5). doi: 10.1080/00045608.2012.687349.

Kwan, M.P. (2018). The neighborhood effect averaging problem (NEAP): An elusive confounder of the neighborhood effect. *International Journal of Environmental Research and Public Health*, 15(9). doi: 10.3390/ijerph15091841.

Laatikainen, T.E., Hasanzadeh, K., Kyttä, M. (2018). Capturing exposure in environmental health research: Challenges and opportunities of different activity space models. *International Journal of Health Geographics*. doi: 10.1186/s12942-018-0149-5.

Leal, C. and Chaix, B. (2011). The influence of geographic life environments on cardiometabolic risk factors: A systematic review, a methodological assessment and a research agenda. *Obesity Reviews*, 12(3), 217–230. doi: 10.1111/j.1467-789X.2010.00726.x.

Lebel, A., Kestens, Y., Pampalon, R., Thériault, M., Daniel, M., Subramanian, S.V. (2012). Local context influence, activity space, and foodscape exposure in two Canadian metropolitan settings: Is daily mobility exposure associated with overweight? *Journal of Obesity*. doi: 10.1155/2012/912645.

Lee, J.H., Davis, A.W., Yoon, S.Y., Goulias, K.G. (2016). Activity space estimation with longitudinal observations of social media data. *Transportation*, 43(6). doi: 10.1007/s11116-016-9719-1.

Letellier, N., Carrière, I., Gutierrez, L.-A., Gabelle, A., Dartigues, J.-F., Dufouil, C., Helmer, C., Cadot, E., Berr, C. (2019). Influence of activity space on the association between neighborhood characteristics and dementia risk: Results from the 3-City study cohort. *BMC Geriatrics*, 19(1). doi:10.1186/s12877-018-1017-7.

Lewin, K. (1936). A dynamic theory of personality. *The Journal of Nervous and Mental Disease*, 85(5), 612–613. doi: 10.1097/00005053-193611000-00051.

Li, J. and Kim, C. (2020). Exploring relationships of grocery shopping patterns and healthy food accessibility in residential neighborhoods and activity space. *Applied Geography*, 116. doi: 10.1016/j.apgeog.2020.102169.

Li, J., Kim, C., Sang, S. (2018). Exploring impacts of land use characteristics in residential neighborhood and activity space on non-work travel behaviors. *Journal of Transport Geography*, 70. doi: 10.1016/j.jtrangeo.2018.06.001.

Lieze, M., Jelle, V.C., Benedicte, D., Nico, V. de W., Mario, M., Van Dyck, D. (2020). Using virtual reality to investigate physical environmental factors related to cycling in older adults: A comparison between two methodologies. *Journal of Transport and Health*, 19. doi: 10.1016/j.jth.2020.100921.

Lipperman-Kreda, S., Finan, L.J., Kowitt, S.D., Grube, J.W., Abadi, M., Balassone, A., Kaner, E. (2020). Youth daily exposure to tobacco outlets and cigarette smoking behaviors: Does exposure within activity space matter? *Addiction*, 115(9). doi: 10.1111/add.15001.

Liu, B., Widener, M., Burgoine, T., Hammond, D. (2020). Association between time-weighted activity space-based exposures to fast food outlets and fast food consumption among young adults in urban Canada. *International Journal of Behavioral Nutrition and Physical Activity*. doi: 10.1186/s12966-020-00967-y.

Ma, X., Li, X., Kwan, M.P., Chai, Y. (2020). Who could not avoid exposure to high levels of residence-based pollution by daily mobility? Evidence of air pollution exposure from the perspective of the neighborhood effect averaging problem (NEAP). *International Journal of Environmental Research and Public Health*, 17(4). doi: 10.3390/ijerph17041223.

Mackett, R.L. (2003). Why do people use their cars for short trips? *Transportation*, 30(3), 329–349. doi: 10.1023/A:1023987812020.

Mason, M., Mennis, J., Way, T., Light, J., Rusby, J., Westling, E., Crewe, S., Flay, B., Campbell, L., Zaharakis, N. et al. (2015). "Young adolescents" perceived activity space risk, peer networks, and substance use. *Health and Place*, 34. doi: 10.1016/j.healthplace.2015.04.005.

Matthews, S.A. (2011). Spatial polygamy and the heterogeneity of place: Studying people and place via egocentric methods. *Communities, Neighborhoods, and Health*. doi: 10.1007/978-1-4419-7482-2_3.

Matthews, S.A. and Yang, T.C. (2013). Spatial polygamy and contextual exposures (SPACEs): Promoting activity space approaches in research on place and health. *American Behavioral Scientist*, 57(8). doi: 10.1177/0002764213487345.

McBride, E.C., Davis, A.W., Goulias, K.G. (2019). Fragmentation in daily schedule of activities using activity sequences. *Transportation Research Record*. doi: 10.1177/0361198119837501.

Meegan, R. and Mitchell, A. (2001). "It's not community round here, it's neighbourhood": Neighbourhood change and cohesion in urban regeneration policies. *Urban Studies*, 38(12). doi: 10.1080/00420980120087117.

Mennis, J., Mason, M., Ambrus, A. (2018). Urban greenspace is associated with reduced psychological stress among adolescents: A geographic ecological momentary assessment (GEMA) analysis of activity space. *Landscape and Urban Planning*, 174. doi: 10.1016/j.landurbplan.2018.02.008.

Miller, H. (2007). Place-based versus people-based geographic information science. *Geography Compass*, 1(3). doi: 10.1111/j.1749-8198.2007.00025.x.

Naud, A., Sueur, C., Chaix, B., Yan, K. (2020). Combining social network and activity space data for health research: Tools and methods. *Health and Place*, 66. doi: 10.1016/j.healthplace.2020.102454.

Perchoux, C. (2015). Accounting for residential and non-residential environments to measure contextual effects on health behavior: The case of recreational walking behavior. PhD Thesis, Université Pierre et Marie Curie-Paris VI/École de santé publique de l'Université de Montréal, Paris/Montreal.

Perchoux, C., Chaix, B., Cummins, S., Kestens, Y. (2013). Conceptualization and measurement of environmental exposure in epidemiology: Accounting for activity space related to daily mobility. *Health and Place*, 21, 86–93. doi:10.1016/j.healthplace.2013.01.005.

Perchoux, C., Kestens, Y., Thomas, F., Hulst, A.V., Thierry, B., Chaix, B. (2014). Assessing patterns of spatial behavior in health studies: Their socio-demographic determinants and associations with transportation modes (the RECORD Cohort Study). *Social Science and Medicine*, 119, 64–73. doi: 10.1016/j.socscimed.2014.07.026.

Perchoux, C., Kestens, Y., Brondeel, R., Chaix, B. (2015). Accounting for the daily locations visited in the study of the built environment correlates of recreational walking (the RECORD Cohort Study). *Preventive Medicine*, 81, 142–149. doi: 10.1016/j.ypmed.2015.08.010.

Perchoux, C., Chaix, B., Brondeel, R., Kestens, Y. (2016). Residential buffer, perceived neighborhood, and individual activity space: New refinements in the definition of exposure areas – The RECORD Cohort Study. *Health and Place*, 40, 116–122. doi: 10.1016/j.healthplace.2016.05.004.

Perchoux, C., Chaix, B., Kestens, Y. (2019a). Activity spaces in place and health research: Novel exposure measures, data collection tools, and designs. *Health and Place*, 58, 102130. doi: 10.1016/j.healthplace.2019.05.008.

Perchoux, C., Brondeel, R., Wasfi, R., Klein, O., Caruso, G., Vallée, J., Klein, S., Thierry, B., Dijst, M., Chaix, B. (2019b). Walking, trip purpose, and exposure to multiple environments: A case study of older adults in Luxembourg. *Journal of Transport and Health*, 13, 170–184. doi: 10.1016/j.jth.2019.04.002.

Plue, R., Jewett, L., Widener, M.J. (2020). Considerations when using individual GPS data in food environment research: A scoping review of "Selective (Daily) Mobility bias" in GPS exposure studies and its relevance to the retail food environment. doi: 10.1007/978-3-030-19573-1_6.

Raskind, I.G., Kegler, M.C., Girard, A.W., Dunlop, A.L., Kramer, M.R. (2020). An activity space approach to understanding how food access is associated with dietary intake and BMI among urban, low-income African American women. *Health and Place*, 66. doi:10.1016/j.healthplace.2020.102458.

Reginster, I. and Edwards, G. (2001). The concept and implementation of perceptual regions as hierarchical spatial units for evaluating environmental sensitivity. *URISA Journal*, 13(1), 5–16.

Robinson, A.I. and Oreskovic, N.M. (2013). Comparing self-identified and census-defined neighborhoods among adolescents using GPS and accelerometer. *International Journal of Health Geographics*, 12. doi: 10.1186/1476-072X-12-57.

Schipperijn, J., Ejstrud, B., Troelsen, J. (2013). GIS: A spatial turn in the health science? *Neighbourhood Structure and Health Promotion*. doi: 10.1007/978-1-4614-6672-7_8.

Schönfelder, S. and Axhausen, K.W. (2003). Activity spaces: Measures of social exclusion? *Transport Policy*, 10(4), 273–286. doi: 10.1016/j.tranpol.2003.07.002.

Scully, J.Y., Moudon, A.V., Hurvitz, P.M., Aggarwal, A., Drewnowski, A. (2017). GPS or travel diary: Comparing spatial and temporal characteristics of visits to fast food restaurants and supermarkets. *PLoS ONE*, 12(4). doi: 10.1371/journal.pone.0174859.

Scully, J.Y., Moudon, A.V., Hurvitz, P.M., Aggarwal, A., Drewnowski, A. (2019). A time-based objective measure of exposure to the food environment. *International Journal of Environmental Research and Public Health*, 16(7), 1180. doi: 10.3390/ijerph16071180.

Shareck, M., Kestens, Y., Gauvin, L. (2013). Examining the spatial congruence between data obtained with a novel activity location questionnaire, continuous GPS tracking, and prompted recall surveys. *International Journal of Health Geographics*, 12(1), 40. doi: 10.1186/1476-072X-12-40.

Shareck, M., Kestens, Y., Vallée, J., Datta, G., Frohlich, K.L. (2016). The added value of accounting for activity space when examining the association between tobacco retailer availability and smoking among young adults. *Tobacco Control*, 25(4). doi: 10.1136/tobaccocontrol-2014-052194.

Shareck, M., Datta, G.D., Vallée, J., Kestens, Y., Frohlich, K.L. (2020). Is smoking cessation in young adults associated with tobacco retailer availability in their activity space? *Nicotine & Tobacco Research: Official Journal of the Society for Research on Nicotine and Tobacco*, 22(4). doi: 10.1093/ntr/nty242.

Sharp, G. and Kimbro, R.T. (2021). Neighborhood social environments, healthy resources, and adult diabetes: Accounting for activity space exposures. *Health and Place*, 67. doi: 10.1016/j.healthplace.2020.102473.

Sharp, G., Denney, J.T., Kimbro, R.T. (2015). Multiple contexts of exposure: Activity spaces, residential neighborhoods, and self-rated health. *Social Science and Medicine*, 146. doi: 10.1016/j.socscimed.2015.10.040.

Sherman, J.E., Spencer, J., Preisser, J.S., Gesler, W.M., Arcury, T.A. (2005). A suite of methods for representing activity space in a healthcare accessibility study. *International Journal of Health Geographics*, 4. doi: 10.1186/1476-072X-4-24.

Shrestha, S., Kestens, Y., Thomas, F., El Aarbaoui, T., Chaix, B. (2019). Spatial access to sport facilities from the multiple places visited and sport practice: Assessing and correcting biases related to selective daily mobility. *Social Science and Medicine*, 236. doi: 10.1016/j.socscimed.2019.112406.

Sloan, L. and Morgan, J. (2015). Who tweets with their location? Understanding the relationship between demographic characteristics and the use of geoservices and geotagging on Twitter. *PLoS ONE*, 10(11). doi: 10.1371/journal.pone.0142209.

Smith, L., Foley, L. Panter, J. (2019). Activity spaces in studies of the environment and physical activity: A review and synthesis of implications for causality. *Health and Place*. doi: 10.17863/CAM.38880.

Stalvey, B.T., Owsley, C., Sloane, M.E., Ball, K. (1999). The life space questionnaire: A measure of the extent of mobility of older adults. *Journal of Applied Gerontology*, 18(4). doi: 10.1177/073346489901800404.

Sturge, J., Klaassens, M., Lager, D., Weitkamp, G., Vegter, D., Meijering, L. (2020). Using the concept of activity space to understand the social health of older adults living with memory problems and dementia at home. *Social Science and Medicine*. doi: 10.1016/j.socscimed.2020.113208.

Susser, M. and Susser, E. (1996). Choosing a future for epidemiology: I. Eras and paradigms. *American Journal of Public Health*, 86(5). doi: 10.2105/AJPH.86.5.668.

Tamura, K., Elbel, B., Chaix, B., Regan, S.D., Al-Ajlouni, Y.A., Athens, J.K., Meline, J., Duncan, D.T. (2017). Residential and GPS-defined activity space neighborhood noise complaints, body mass index and blood pressure among low-income housing residents in New York City. *Journal of Community Health*, 42(5). doi: 10.1007/s10900-017-0344-5.

Tamura, K., Elbel, B., Athens, J.K., Rummo, P.E., Chaix, B., Regan, S.D., Al-Ajlouni, Y.A., Duncan, D.T. (2018). Assessments of residential and global positioning system activity space for food environments, body mass index and blood pressure among low-income housing residents in New York City. *Geospatial Health*, 13(2). doi: 10.4081/gh.2018.712.

Thierry, B., Chaix, B., Kestens, Y. (2013). Detecting activity locations from raw GPS data: A novel kernel-based algorithm. *International Journal of Health Geographics*, 12(14). doi: 10.1186/1476-072X-12-14.

Tindall, D.B. and Wellman, B. (2001). Canada as social structure: Social network analysis and Canadian sociology. *Canadian Journal of Sociology*, 265–308. doi: 10.2307/3341889.

Traoré, M., Vallée, J., Chauvin, P. (2020). Risk of late cervical cancer screening in the Paris region according to social deprivation and medical densities in daily visited neighborhoods. *International Journal of Health Geographics*, 19(1). doi: 10.1186/s12942-020-00212-6.

Tribby, C.P., Miller, H.J., Brown, B.B., Werner, C.M., Smith, K.R. (2015). Assessing built environment walkability using activity-space summary measures. *Journal of Transport and Land Use*. doi: 10.5198/jtlu.2015.625.

Vallée, J. (2021). La force des lieux faibles. *PasserelleSHS*, 1. doi: 10.48649/pshs.91.

Vallée, J. and Chauvin, P. (2012). Investigating the effects of medical density on health-seeking behaviours using a multiscale approach to residential and activity spaces: Results from a prospective cohort study in the Paris metropolitan area, France. *International Journal of Health Geographics*, 11. doi: 10.1186/1476-072X-11-54.

Vallée, J., Cadot, E., Grillo, F., Parizot, I., Chauvin, P. (2010). The combined effects of activity space and neighbourhood of residence on participation in preventive healthcare activities: The case of cervical screening in the Paris metropolitan area (France). *Health and Place*, 16(5). doi: 10.1016/j.healthplace.2010.04.009.

Vallée, J., Cadot, E., Roustit, C., Parizot, I., Chauvin, P. (2011). The role of daily mobility in mental health inequalities: The interactive influence of activity space and neighbourhood of residence on depression. *Social Science and Medicine*, 73(8), 1133–1144. doi: 10.1016/j.socscimed.2011.08.009.

Vallée, J., Commenges, H., Perchoux, C., Kestens, Y. (2015). Mobilité quotidienne et accès potentiel aux ressources urbaines en Île-de-France : quelles inégalités sociales ? *Données urbaines 7*, 87–95.

Wang, J., Kwan, M.P., Chai, Y. (2018). An innovative context-based crystal-growth activity space method for environmental exposure assessment: A study using GIS and GPS trajectory data collected in Chicago. *International Journal of Environmental Research and Public Health*, 15(4). doi: 10.3390/ijerph15040703.

Widener, M.J., Minaker, L.M., Reid, J.L., Patterson, Z., Ahmadi, T.K., Hammond, D. (2018). Activity space-based measures of the food environment and their relationships to food purchasing behaviours for young urban adults in Canada. *International Journal of Middle East Studies*, 21(11). doi: 10.1017/S1368980018000435.

Wolpert, J. (1965). Behavioral aspects of the decision to migrate. *Papers of the Regional Science Association*, 15(1). doi: 10.1007/BF01947871.

Worrell, M.C., Kramer, M., Yamin, A., Ray, S.M., Goswami, N.D. (2017). Use of activity space in a tuberculosis outbreak: Bringing homeless persons into spatial analyses. *Open Forum Infectious Diseases*, 4(1). doi: 10.1093/ofid/ofw280.

Zenk, S.N., Schulz, A.J., Matthews, S.A., Odoms-Young, A., Wilbur, J.E., Wegrzyn, L., Gibbs, K., Braunschweig, C., Stokes, C. (2011). Activity space environment and dietary and physical activity behaviors: A pilot study. *Health and Place*, 17(5). doi: 10.1016/j.healthplace.2011.05.001.

Zenk, S.N., Matthews, S.A., Kraft, A.N., Jones, K.K. (2018). How many days of global positioning system (GPS) monitoring do you need to measure activity space environments in health research? *Health and Place*, 51. doi: 10.1016/j.healthplace.2018.02.004.

Zenk, S.N., Kraft, A.N., Jones, K.K., Matthews, S.A. (2019). Convergent validity of an activity-space survey for use in health research. *Health and Place*, 56. doi: 10.1016/j.healthplace.2019.01.009.

Zhang, L., Kwan, M.P., Chen, F., Lin, R., Zhou, S. (2018). Impacts of individual daily greenspace exposure on health based on individual activity space and structural equation modeling. *International Journal of Environmental Research and Public Health*, 15(10). doi: 10.3390/ijerph15102323.

# 3

# Daily Mobility and Social Inequalities in Health: A Conceptual Framework and Application

**Martine SHARECK**
*Université de Sherbrooke, Canada*

## 3.1. Introduction

Researchers studying environmental effects on health are becoming increasingly interested in daily mobility and the activity space (Inagami et al. 2007; Mason and Korpela 2009; Basta et al. 2010; Zenk et al. 2011; Kestens et al. 2012; Shareck et al. 2015; Perchoux et al. 2016), which is defined as "the subset of all locations within which an individual has direct contact as a result of his or her day-to-day activities" (Golledge and Stimson 1997, p. 279).

Around the beginning of the 2000s, criticisms were raised as to the focus hitherto placed almost exclusively on the neighborhood of residence as the most relevant living environment for studying health and social inequalities in health. These criticisms were part of the mobility turn observed in the social sciences (Sheller and Urry 2006) and became manifest in the call to adopt a relational approach to place (Cummins et al. 2007), to develop more personalized environmental exposure measurements (Kwan 2009) and to overcome the "local trap" (Cummins 2007) or the "residential trap" (Chaix

*Everyday Mobility and Health*,
coordinated by Julie VALLÉE. 

et al. 2009). Although many studies have looked into the relationship between daily mobility, the environment and health, few of them have focused on *social inequalities in health,* that is, the gaps in health between different social groups. This is so despite the fact that as several authors have pointed out, daily mobility is a central driver of social stratification and inequality (Kaufmann et al. 2004; Jiron 2007; Manderscheid 2009).

Numerous studies have demonstrated that social inequalities in the characteristics of the neighborhood of residence – defined as physical attributes (such as green spaces, food shops, health services, air pollution) and social attributes (e.g. level of deprivation, social cohesion, crime rate) of neighborhoods – could lead to health inequalities (Kawachi and Berkman 2003; Riva et al. 2007). Considering this, it is also plausible for inequalities in the exposures experienced during commuting and day-to-day activities to have an influence on social inequalities in health. On the one hand, the amenities, services and environmental characteristics that support social inclusion and shape health are unevenly distributed across space (Golledge and Stimson 1997). On the other hand, the places in which various social groups conduct their daily activities may be limited due to social structure, including class and power relations (Hägerstrand 1970; Gatrell 2002). It therefore seems relevant to take daily mobility into account when addressing social inequalities in health.

This chapter will introduce a conceptual framework to reflect on the links between social inequalities in daily mobility and social inequalities in health (Shareck et al. 2014a). Social inequalities in health will be defined in section 3.2, followed by a presentation of the conceptual framework (section 3.3), built on the basis of empirical data describing social inequalities in relation to two dimensions of daily mobility:

– the extent to which one is (im)mobile;

– the characteristics of the places visited and the amenities and services encountered during daily travel and activities.

Section 3.3.4 will describe the mechanisms through which social inequalities in daily mobility can contribute to social inequalities in health. We will then apply the conceptual framework to a contemporary issue, the Covid-19 pandemic (section 3.4), in order to illustrate the way in which mobility and the activity locations of more or less marginalized groups could put them at risk of contracting the disease, or suffering from the pandemic's psychosocial and collateral impacts. Section 3.5 will conclude with a brief discussion on some practical implications of the conceptual framework for creating healthy and equitable cities.

## 3.2. Social inequalities in health: definition, extent and progression

We define social inequalities in health as systematic differences in the health states or behaviors of groups occupying unequal positions in the social hierarchy due to their wealth, power, race or any other dimension of dominance or marginalization (Braveman 2006). Social stratification variables, which shape the uneven distribution of disease and health across the population, include income, education, employment and housing conditions, as well as belonging to groups prone to discrimination due to ethno-cultural background, gender or physical disability (Frohlich and De Koninck 2008; World Health Organization 2008).

The portrait of social inequalities in health varies across cities, regions and countries as well as over time, depending on the chosen health and social indicators. Here, we do not intend to provide a thorough portrait of social inequalities in health. However, it is relevant to note that social inequalities have been documented for a range of health indicators such as life expectancy, morbidity and mortality, perceived physical and mental health, well-being, smoking, alcohol consumption, physical activity, food and the use of healthcare services (Frohlich and De Koninck 2008).

In general, the health of the population has tended to improve over recent decades, not only among more advantaged groups but also among the less advantaged groups (Frohlich and De Koninck 2008). The upward trend in life expectancy and in healthy life expectancy has nonetheless been curbed by Covid-19 in several countries worldwide (Andrasfay and Goldman 2021; Woolf et al. 2021). For their part, social inequalities in health have tended to widen, with the health of more advantaged groups improving more markedly than that of less advantaged groups (Frohlich and De Koninck 2008; Marmot et al. 2020a); this has become even more pronounced since the onset of the pandemic in 2020 (Marmot et al. 2020b). Bearing this in mind, it becomes all the more urgent to better appraise how our daily activities and living environments influence social inequalities in health, with a view to implementing interventions and policies in order to reduce them.

## 3.3. Conceptual framework

The conceptual framework draws on health and social geography, health promotion, sociology, urban studies and transportation research. In general, a conceptual framework is essential for testing research hypotheses developed a priori, and for preventing the post-hoc theorization of causal links. This avoids (over)interpreting empirical results based on assumptions, facilitates the replication of studies in various contexts and contributes to the creation of a rigorous and unified body of knowledge (Frohlich et al. 2004).

In relation to the central theme of this chapter, this conceptual framework will be useful for analyzing and understanding the links between daily mobility and social inequalities in health in a systematic, comprehensive and nuanced manner.

We succinctly conceptualize the links between daily mobility and social inequalities in health as being anchored in the concept of "mobility potential". Mobility potential is defined as the "ability to move through geographic and social space", and represents an unevenly distributed resource among social groups (Kaufmann et al. 2004, p. 750). Mobility potential is transformed into "effective mobility", or what are also called "mobility patterns", via individual agency.

Several effective mobility indicators exist, two of which are an integral part of this conceptual framework:

– the fact of moving or not (i.e. (im)mobility);

– the contextual exposures arising from this (im)mobility.

Social inequalities in mobility potential and in effective mobility may lead to social inequalities in health. The concepts of mobility potential, individual agency and effective mobility can be considered as anchored in a social context (Camarero and Oliva 2008; Kaufmann 2011; Manderscheid 2014) involving social norms and structures such as class, gender and race structures (Poland et al. 2006). In that sense, daily mobility is not a purely individual attribute, but rather relates to the interaction between an individual and the context in which they evolve. These concepts, their operationalization and their interrelationships will be described below.

### 3.3.1. *Daily mobility potential: an unevenly distributed resource*

The concept of mobility potential is the range of travel options available to individuals. Can individuals move or not? If they can, by what means(s)? What are the characteristics of all the places, amenities and services they can choose from to perform an activity or meet a given need?

The concept of mobility potential was originally proposed by Kaufmann et al. (2004) to conceptualize the link between spatial mobility and social inequality, for example in terms of unequal access to safe and quality jobs based on poverty level, gender or physical disability. It makes it possible to better understand the underlying causes for daily mobility differences between social groups (Camarero and Oliva 2008). Mobility potential also makes room for the individual as an agent of change. This particular trait addresses the criticisms mentioned in the introduction, namely the need to acknowledge the individual in the definition of space, having an influence on health and the resulting environmental exposures (Cummins et al. 2007; Kwan 2009).

The few attempts to operationalize mobility potential have generally been limited to describing one's access to different modes of transport (e.g. the car) and the physical capacity of individuals to use various modes of transport to move through space (Flamm and Kaufmannn 2006; Shin 2011). Little attention has been given to potentially accessible locations, amenities and services while remaining (im)mobile (Jiron 2007) although, as has been pointed out (Urry 2007, p. 187): "social inequalities cannot be reduced merely by improving access to the means of mobilities. What is at stake are the activities, values and goods to which mobilities allow access".

The concept of mobility potential is interesting for the study of social inequalities in health because it is shaped both by individual characteristics (such as preferences, needs, modes of transport), social characteristics (such as gender, income, level of education, ethnicity) and a person's geographical circumstances (e.g. the proximity to certain places of activity, amenities and services the individual might wish to access from the place of residence) (Kaufmannn et al. 2004; Manderscheid 2009). It is also shaped by conditions or "authority constraints" which Hägerstrand describes as "the general rules, laws, economic barriers and power relations which determine who has or does not have access to specific places at specific times" (Pred 1977, p. 208). These conditions may include pricing and rights mechanisms (Golledge and Stimson 1997; Bernard et al. 2007), as well as social norms (Jiron 2007;

Reynolds 2013; Skelton 2013). These individual, social and geographical characteristics – as well as the rules governing access to places, amenities and services – are considered fundamentally related to the larger societal context, in other words, to the social, cultural, economic and political structures in which mobility is actualized (Kaufmannn et al. 2004, p. 750). Because of this, we can expect the emergence of inequalities in the potential for mobility and, as a consequence, in the effective mobility of different social groups (Kaufmannn et al. 2004, 2018; Weiss 2005; Manderscheid 2009).

Furthermore, individual, social and geographical characteristics, as well as access rules, interact with one another to allow or hinder the mobility possibilities of certain social groups. For example, due to an interaction between personal income and price, certain goods, such as healthy foods, which are usually priced higher than unhealthy foods, are less accessible to less fortunate groups. An additional constraint could be related to the mobility potential of less fortunate groups, which may be limited by the cost of traveling to access healthy foods at lower prices than the ones available near their place of residence.

Social and civic rights are another type of condition determining access to the services offered by formal (and often State-funded) institutions (Bernard et al. 2007). For example, in Quebec, access to municipal libraries or to public health or employment assistance services may be reserved for specific populations, depending on their place of residence, age, employment status or income. This is the case with certain front-line healthcare services administered by the public system that are intended for residents of a specific catchment area, based on priority. On a similar note, the geographic distribution of amenities, services and features of the physical environment is neither socially nor politically neutral (Harvey 1973; Soja 2010). For example, public transport and bike paths may not be evenly or equitably distributed across space (Miciukiewicz and Vigar 2012), although this may depend on a city's urban planning policies (Fuller et al. 2013). Another example involves teenagers from less affluent backgrounds who may not attend recreational facilities or renowned schools in affluent neighborhoods due to unwritten rules conveying that they are not welcome there, or because they feel "out of place". Their mobility potential would exclude these amenities and services due to a combination of unspoken rules in affluent neighborhoods (social norms, discrimination) and the desire of young people to have a sense of belonging (Skelton 2013).

These few examples illustrate how mobility potential depends on individual, social, geographical characteristics, as well as access rules. They prove that the facilities, amenities, goods and services promoting health are not evenly or equitably available to all. As it intrinsically incorporates the idea that social factors determine the universe of mobility possibilities one can (or is forced to) choose from, the concept of mobility potential is useful for recognizing the existence of social inequalities in mobility (Hägerstrand 1970) and for better understanding their impact on social inequalities in health.

### 3.3.2. *Converting mobility potential into effective mobility: the role of individual agency*

Mobility potential is converted into effective mobility through individual agency (Kaufmannn et al. 2004; Weiss 2005; Jiron 2007; Manderscheid 2009). We define individual agency as the ability "to intervene in the world, or to refrain from such intervention, with the effect of influencing a specific process or state of affairs" (Giddens 1984, p. 14). As emphasized in Sen's (1999) capability approach, individual agency is expressed in a social context and reflects a person's ability to choose from the range of options available to them to engage in the activities they value. In the present case, this is translated as a person's ability to choose from available mobility options – including the option of whether or not to move, as well as where to go – and to actualize that choice (Kaufmannn et al. 2004; Manderscheid 2009).

For example, a person can *choose* to move outside their neighborhood of residence to go shopping at their favorite shop, or they can *be forced* to travel long distances in order to access goods and services not readily available near their place of residence. Conversely, someone may choose to concentrate their activities near their place of residence provided that everyday needs can be met nearby, or they may be forced to stay in the area if physical or social constraints hinder mobility, or if the required modes of transport are unavailable.

It should be noted that individual agency is shaped by individual, social and geographic factors as well as by conditions similar to those influencing mobility potential. This implies that differences in individual agency between social groups may exist. The links between daily mobility and social inequalities in health may derive from the joint contribution of inequalities in individual agency and mobility potential, rather than from one explanation or the other (Abel and Frohlich 2012).

For example, several reasons could explain why low-income groups are more at risk of having an unhealthy diet: their limited economic means compared to the higher price of healthy food (inequalities in individual socio-economic resources), a lower availability of fresh fruit and vegetable shops near their place of residence and a mobility potential limited by the traveling costs for gaining access to healthy food at lower prices than the food available near their place of residence (inequalities in terms of mobility potential), as well as a lesser ability to transform their mobility potential for taking advantage of other food resources (e.g. food banks) located in their neighborhood (inequalities in terms of individual agency).

By integrating individual agency, the conceptual framework allows us to go beyond determinism (both individual and environmental) and to produce more nuanced hypotheses and explanations regarding the links between the environment and social inequalities in health.

### 3.3.3. *Effective mobility: daily mobility patterns*

By turning our attention towards effective mobility and daily mobility patterns, we shift from what people have the *potential to do* to what they *actually do*. Mobility patterns are directly related to mobility potential: social differences in effective mobility reflect social differences in the characteristics, circumstances and conditions shaping mobility potential as well as social differences in individual agency. We posit that daily mobility patterns are structured by key locations such as the place of residence, workplace or place of study (Golledge and Stimson 1997). These comprise spatial and temporal dimensions and include whether or not to move, spatial extent, the degree of constraint, flexibility and spontaneity of movements, the types of activities performed, as well as the characteristics of the places in which activities are carried out, not to mention the amenities and services encountered while traveling (Ramadier et al. 2005).

Our conceptual framework emphasizes two dimensions of effective mobility:

– whether to move or not;

– the characteristics of the activity places and amenities/services found during daily travel, also known as "contextual exposures".

These two dimensions of daily mobility are the ones that have attracted the most interest in studies on social inequalities in health.

For example, empirical studies have found that lower income groups are more likely to travel shorter distances to carry out daily activities compared to higher income groups (Gough 2008; Vallée et al. 2010; Morency et al. 2011), although this observation may depend on urban planning (Schönfelder and Axhausen 2003). Compared to other occupational groups, students or full-time workers tend to travel greater distances daily (Paez et al. 2010; Morency et al. 2011), whereas part-time workers and the unemployed are more likely to limit their activities to the area surrounding their place of residence (Kwan 2000; Vallée et al. 2010; Zenk et al. 2011). Individuals' education level has also been associated with daily mobility patterns: less educated groups tend to travel less than more educated groups (Golledge and Stimson 1997; Vallée et al. 2010; Shareck et al. 2014b). While the possession of a driver's license, a personal vehicle, a monthly transit pass or a car-sharing subscription would promote mobility (Kaufmannn et al. 2004; Naess 2006; Casas 2007; Frandberg and Vilhelmson 2011; Morency et al. 2011; Zenk et al. 2011), expenses relating to the distances traveled to gain access to certain services might dissuade people from doing so (Gough 2008; Skelton 2013). The environmental characteristics of the neighborhood of residence such as the level of deprivation (Shareck et al. 2014b) or the density of destinations have also been associated with distinct mobility patterns (Kestens et al. 2010).

Although this way of operationalizing daily mobility (i.e., depending on whether one travels or not, and the distances covered) is considered essential for access to work, education, health and leisure (Miciukiewicz and Vigar 2012), and more broadly, to social inclusion (Stanley et al. 2011) and well-being (Spinney et al. 2009), it has hardly been taken into account in the literature. However, here again it is important to consider the characteristics of the places, amenities and services available while traveling (or not). Social inequalities have been documented in this regard, particularly in relation to a person's social role (e.g. gender) (Gough 2008; Kwan 2000; Shin 2011; Shareck et al. 2014b; Kim and Kwan 2021), social position (e.g. income, education or occupation) (Kestens et al. 2010; Paez et al. 2010, p. 201; Christian 2012; Shareck et al. 2014b; Krivo et al. 2013; Kim and

Kwan 2021) or relationships with others (e.g. social networks) (McPherson et al. 2001; Matthews et al. 2005; Skelton 2013).

For example, American and Canadian studies have noted that people with lower levels of education tend to conduct daily activities in more disadvantaged neighborhoods or closer to tobacco retailers (Shareck et al. 2015, 2018a) compared to their more educated counterparts (Krivo et al. 2013; Shareck et al. 2014b). Studies have also suggested that residents of deprived neighborhoods encounter a larger density of convenience stores and fast-food restaurants during their daily commute, compared to residents of more affluent neighborhoods (Kestens et al. 2010). In another study, women encountered fewer educational, employment and leisure opportunities during their daily commute than men (Kwan 2000). Similarly, a study from the UK suggested that children from more deprived neighborhoods were more often exposed, and exposed for longer, to tobacco retailers during their daily activities compared to young people from more affluent neighborhoods (Caryl et al. 2020). Finally, qualitative studies have shown that implicit rules can govern whether social groups are welcome (or not) in specific places and have access (or not) to certain amenities and services (White and Green 2011; Reynolds 2013). For example, a study of African diaspora youth living in a deprived area of London, UK, revealed that many school children preferred to attend schools located in their area (even if these were less reputable), because they did not feel they belonged to privileged schools located outside their neighborhood (Reynolds 2013). These few examples illustrate the social gaps that can exist in the quality of places, amenities and services encountered during daily travel.

### 3.3.4. *From daily mobility to social inequalities in health*

Our conceptual framework can help to identify different mechanisms through which social inequalities in daily mobility could lead to social inequalities in health. We will present them below. According to our conceptual framework, the link between daily mobility and social inequalities in health depends on several factors such as:

– whether mobility is restricted and the characteristics of the environment where restricted mobility takes place;

– the combination of residential and activity space exposures;

– whether mobility occurs between environments that share similar characteristics or not.

#### 3.3.4.1. *Daily mobility limited to the neighborhood of residence*

A first mechanism involves mobility that is limited to the neighborhood of residence. This can directly influence health in a positive or negative way. Restricted daily travel can lead to social exclusion by limiting access to employment opportunities and quality education, health and leisure services (Preston and Rajé 2007; Stanley et al. 2011). Furthermore, this can influence health by delaying access to medical consultations, for example (Vallée et al. 2010). However, the effects of restricted mobility on health and social health inequalities greatly depend on the characteristics of the environment an individual is confined to. While restricted mobility could be detrimental to the health of residents of socially disadvantaged neighborhoods (or neighborhoods poor in health-promoting resources), it could have null to positive effects on the health of residents of better-off neighborhoods (and those areas better equipped with health-promoting amenities and services). This differential effect related to neighborhood characteristics was observed in a study by Vallée et al. (2011) who found that among participants who concentrated their daily activities in their neighborhood of residence, those who lived in affluent neighborhoods had better mental health than those in more disadvantaged neighborhoods (Vallée et al. 2011). Other authors have noted an interactive effect between the individual socio-economic level and that of the neighborhood. This interaction means that living in an affluent neighborhood when we are ourselves disadvantaged may be harmful for creating and maintaining a social network and for well-being, whereas living in a less affluent neighborhood but being better-off ourselves may promote the creation of social ties and well-being (Browne-Yung et al. 2013).

Whether restricted mobility is *constrained* or *chosen* may also have a differential impact on health. In fact, living in a neighborhood in which we can find all the resources and services needed to function on a daily basis reduces the need for traveling. In this case, an individual may choose to limit their mobility, and the simple fact of having the choice may benefit their health. On the other hand, being confined to a neighborhood despite the desire to move around could be detrimental to health, regardless of the neighborhood's characteristics. This is where individual agency comes into play, by turning mobility potential into effective mobility (see section 3.3.2). When looking at the links between daily mobility and social inequalities in health, it is essential to not only dwell on the characteristics of the places in which restricted mobility occurs, but also to understand why the mobility of certain groups is more restricted than that of others, and in particular whether this stems from a free choice or a constraint.

### 3.3.4.2. *Daily mobility beyond the neighborhood of residence*

Daily mobility limited to the neighborhood of residence has generally been associated with social exclusion and adverse health effects, although the previous section suggests that this hypothesis needs to be nuanced. Similarly, some authors have suggested that its corollary (high and extended mobility regardless of the destination) increases access to amenities and services while promoting social inclusion and health (Stanley et al. 2011; Allen and Hollingworth 2013). In an Australian study, high mobility – expressed by the number of trips and activities carried out over a given period – was associated with a reduction in the risk of social exclusion, measured by an index combining household income, employment status, social participation and social support, thus improving well-being (Stanley et al. 2011).

However, several authors have pointed out that mobility itself does not necessarily involve social inclusion and health (Cass et al. 2005). Time spent commuting can actually reduce the time available to engage in other health-enhancing activities such as hobbies, or to access quality amenities and services, whether offered locally or not (Jiron 2007). High mobility is in fact not always a sign of wealth or privilege but sometimes illustrates a necessity (Delbosc and Currie 2011). For example, residents of neighborhoods with no healthy food stores or recreational facilities may have to travel long distances to access those health-promoting resources.

In a similar vein, a qualitative study on the daily mobility of residents from Santiago de Chile by Jiron (2007) pointed out that daily commuting time varied considerably from one social group to another, particularly depending on the means of transportation used. The author was able to make a distinction between two groups of workers: those who had a good income but very little free time (the cash-rich, time-poor) and who chose to get to work by car; and those who had a low income but more time to devote to commuting (the cash-poor, time-rich) and who traveled by public transport. This example illustrates how different social groups can have different mobilities depending on their mobility potential, as well as their individual agency and their ability to transform this potential into distinct mobility patterns. Nevertheless, in both groups, the need to travel for work was similarly stressful and detrimental to health and well-being (Jiron 2007).

The examples presented in this section suggest that mobility itself can have both negative and positive health impacts, which depend on a range of circumstances.

### 3.3.4.3. *Characteristics of the activity space*

Another mechanism relating daily mobility to social inequalities in health involves the characteristics of the places visited and that of the amenities and services encountered during daily travel. We will first address the potential links between exposures in the activity space considered as a whole and social inequalities in health. In section 3.4.4, we will discuss the influence that characteristics of the non-residential activity space may have relative to characteristics of the neighborhood of residence.

Studies on health and the characteristics, amenities and services of the activity space have mainly focused on features such as the level of deprivation (Inagami et al. 2007; Sharp et al. 2015; Kimbro et al. 2017), the foodscape (Zenk et al. 2011; Christian 2012; Kestens et al. 2012; Lebel et al. 2012; Clary et al. 2015; Burgoine et al. 2016; Shareck et al. 2018b), green spaces (Zenk et al. 2011; Rodríguez et al. 2012; Bell et al. 2015) and tobacco retailers (Kirchner et al. 2013; Shortt et al. 2014; Lipperman-Kreda et al. 2015; Shareck et al. 2015, 2018a) or alcoholic outlets (Freisthler et al. 2019; Morrison et al. 2019). These characteristics have been studied in relation to health conditions or behaviors such as perceived health (Inagami et al. 2007; Sharp et al. 2015; Kimbro et al. 2017), body mass index (Christian 2012; Clary et al. 2012; Lebel et al. 2012; Burgoine et al. 2016; Kimbro et al. 2017), diabetes (Sharp and Kimbro 2021), the diet ( Zenk et al. 2011; Christian 2012; Shareck et al. 2018b), physical activity (Rodriguez et al. 2012; Zenk et al. 2011), smoking practices (Kirchner et al. 2013; Shortt et al. 2014; Shareck et al. 2015, 2018a) and alcohol consumption (Freisthler et al. 2019; Morrison et al. 2019).

The majority of these studies have not specifically addressed social inequalities in behavior and health conditions. We can nonetheless assume that if certain social groups are excluded from areas of a city or from environments offering a certain type or quality of resources (Krivo et al. 2013; Reynolds 2013; Shareck et al. 2014b), social inequalities in exposures measured in the activity space could ensue and consequently contribute to health inequalities.

For example, a study of young adults in Montreal (Canada) by Shareck et al. (2018) reported that less educated young people lived in neighborhoods and attended places of activity located closer to tobacco retailers, compared to their more educated counterparts. They were also more at risk of being smokers and less likely to quit, which could partly be explained by their greater daily residential and non-residential exposure to tobacco retailers (Shareck et al. 2015, 2018a). Similarly, Burgoine et al. (2016) observed that low-income groups were exposed to a greater number of fast-food restaurants in their activity space (defined as the combination of residential and work neighborhoods), and that this contributed to social inequalities in obesity (Burgoine et al. 2016).

#### 3.3.4.4. *Characteristics of the activity space in relation to those of the residential neighborhood*

The effect of activity space characteristics on social inequalities in health may depend on the relative difference between these and the features of the residential neighborhood, rather than on either of these contexts considered independently (Inagami et al. 2007; Sharp et al. 2015; Kimbro et al. 2017; Sharp and Kimbro 2021); see Chapter 2. For example, two American studies observed that people tended to report poorer perceived health when they frequented neighborhoods with a different level of socio-economic deprivation from that of their residential neighborhood. Residents from socio-economically disadvantaged neighborhoods who worked, studied or spent time in more affluent neighborhoods reported poorer perceived health compared to those who spent time in neighborhoods as poor as theirs (Inagami et al. 2007; Sharp et al. 2015). A parallel can be drawn with a study showing that residents who are themselves socially disadvantaged and who live in affluent neighborhoods can suffer from internalized stigma associated with feeling excluded from amenities and services offered locally (Browne-Yung et al. 2013). Similarly, the conditions of the neighborhood of residence and of the non-residential activity space can exert a compensatory effect on health conditions, such as the risk of diabetes. For example, living in a disadvantaged neighborhood that is associated, in certain studies, with the risk of suffering from diabetes, can be compensated by attending activity places that are well-equipped with amenities and services promoting healthy lifestyles, such as parks and other leisure resources or healthy grocery stores (Sharp and Kimbro 2021).

The example presented in section 3.3 shows that the scenarios arising from the four mechanisms discussed are numerous, but one conclusion can be drawn: the links between daily mobility and social inequalities in health are complex and more nuanced than we might think. It is therefore important to study them in depth, always keeping in mind that daily mobility takes place in a given social and geographic context.

## 3.4. A contemporary example: the Covid-19 pandemic

Let us now apply the conceptual framework to a contemporary public health issue: the Covid-19 pandemic. In many countries, health restrictions enforced to curb the spread of the coronavirus responsible for the Covid-19 pandemic included major restrictions on the daily mobility of entire populations for varying periods of time. In several countries, the political authorities ordered the population to stay at home and to turn to teleworking for an extended period (Ritchie et al. 2020). Often, only essential workers such as those in the health or the agri-food industries maintained their right to travel to work. In some cases, the orders invoked limited non-essential traveling and/or required citizens to travel only near their places of residence. In France, for example, travel was limited to a radius of one kilometer from the place of residence and to one outing taking no longer than one hour at a time. In Quebec and several European countries, a curfew was imposed, prohibiting travel after a certain time of day.

The Covid-19 pandemic example presents two interesting scenarios with regard to our conceptualization of the links between daily (im)mobility and social inequalities in health. On the one hand, restrictions in daily mobility were imposed on the vast majority of the population against their will, and, on the other hand, essential workers were forced to pursue their activities, consequently exposing themselves to an increased risk of contracting the virus. The Covid-19 pandemic highlighted, and even amplified, social and health inequalities that were already evident before the crisis broke out (Bambra et al. 2020; Van Dorn et al. 2020). Inequalities in the experience of public authorities' orders relating to daily commuting, and thus to mobility patterns, both in terms of (im)mobility and the characteristics of the places attended, could have contributed to this.

Concerning the order to limit our daily travel to nearby places, few empirical studies have documented its impact to date. On the other hand, as has been previously discussed, the amenities and services favorable to health such as parks and green spaces, highly coveted in pandemic times, are not always evenly distributed across urban space (Canadian Institute for Health

Information 2011). It is quite plausible for residents of socio-economically disadvantaged neighborhoods and individuals already at higher risk of suffering from the psychosocial impacts of the pandemic – such as those living in substandard or overcrowded housing – to have been more negatively affected by this restriction (Alexander and Shareck 2021). In several Canadian cities, for example, it was observed that at the beginning of the pandemic outdoor physical activity increased more for children and adolescents from wealthier families compared to young people from less affluent families. Similarly, the low residential density and the greater distance from main roads, often characteristic of more affluent neighborhoods, favored outdoor activities. On the other hand, in this same study, high residential density (characterized by the presence of apartment towers) was not necessarily an obstacle to outdoor activities, provided that parks were available nearby (Mitra et al. 2020).

Essential workers, for their part, were exempted from the order to confine themselves. Instead, policy makers encouraged them to pursue their work despite the increased risks of catching and spreading the coronavirus. In several cities around the world, Covid-19 cases were actually concentrated in historically disadvantaged neighborhoods where a high proportion of newcomers lived, in low-income households or in households not speaking the host language (Public Health Ontario 2020), groups that were overrepresented among essential workers and precarious workers who could not turn to teleworking (Berkowitz et al. 2020; Government of Canada 2020a). Despite the order to confine themselves, in general, daily mobility decreased less in those neighborhoods than in more affluent neighborhoods (Weill et al. 2020; Zhai et al. 2021). In addition, residents of more disadvantaged neighborhoods were more likely to visit places (such as food stores), which were smaller and in which the clientele was denser, implying more favorable conditions to virus transmission (Chang et al. 2020).

A Belgian study on the working population also reported an uneven distribution of Covid-19 cases by gender: women being disadvantaged in comparison to men. In this study, these inequalities could be explained by the fact that women had to continue traveling for work in health-related professions, often by public transit (Hawkes and Buse 2020), while continuing to fulfill their family and domestic responsibilities such as food shopping (Ella 2020). Women were not as able as men to limit their daily travel, thus being at a higher risk of coming into contact with the virus. Throughout the pandemic, certain groups who were already socio-economically disadvantaged were therefore more at risk of contracting the disease and spreading it in their living environments due to precarious living and working conditions (Government of Canada 2020b).

## 3.5. Conclusion

In conclusion, mobility is an integral part of our daily lives (Jiron 2007) and, as such, it is fundamental to consider it when studying environmental influences on health. However, not all social groups have the same mobility potential or mobility patterns. Drawing inspiration from conceptual and empirical work carried out in various disciplines of the social sciences and health, we have developed a conceptual framework associating daily mobility with social inequalities in health.

The conceptual proposal is particularly useful for:

– empirically studying the mechanisms through which social inequalities in mobility potential and effective mobility are produced;

– identifying population subgroups which could be "trapped" (due to restricted mobility) in residential neighborhoods with poor amenities and health-promoting services;

– identifying subgroups forced to conduct their daily activities in areas lacking in amenities and health-promoting services;

– better assessing individuals' actual exposure to the resources and characteristics of activity places, and their relationship with health and social inequalities in health (Chaix et al. 2013).

This conceptual proposal may also have implications for urban planning policies and practices. As has already been mentioned, high mobility should not be an end in itself: it does not automatically entail social inclusion, nor does mere attendance at high-quality activity places itself promote health. According to Soja (2010), resources and opportunities will always be somewhat unevenly distributed across space. The simple fact of promoting increased mobility for all might not make it possible to counteract this uneven spatial distribution. We should not neglect the personal and social factors shaping the mobility potential and individual agency, and which therefore contribute to producing and reproducing inequalities in effective mobility. It therefore appears that interventions and policies aimed at creating healthy cities and at reducing social and health inequalities should focus on improving people's mobility potential, as well as their capacity to occupy the places in the city they wish to occupy, both of which are closely linked to social class.

## 3.6. References

Abel, T. and Frohlich, K.L. (2012). Capitals and capabilities: Linking structure and agency to reduce health inequalities. *Soc. Sci. Med.*, 74, 236–244. doi: 10.1016/j.socscimed.2011.10.028.

Alexander, S.A. and Shareck, M. (2021). Widening the gap? Unintended consequences of health promotion measures for young people during COVID-19 lockdown. *Health Promot. Int.* doi: 10.1093/heapro/daab015.

Allen, K. and Hollingworth, S. (2013). "Sticky subjects" or "cosmopolitan creatives"? Social class, place and urban young people's aspirations for work in the knowledge economy. *Urban Stud.*, 50, 499–517. doi: 10.1177/0042098012468901.

Andrasfay, T. and Goldman, N. (2021). Reductions in 2020 US life expectancy due to COVID-19 and the disproportionate impact on the Black and Latino populations. *Proc. Natl. Acad. Sci.*, 118. doi: 10.1073/pnas.2014746118.

Bambra, C., Riordan, R., Ford, J., Matthews, F. (2020). The COVID-19 pandemic and health inequalities. *J. Epidemiol. Community Health.* doi: 10.1136/jech-2020-214401.

Basta, L.A., Richmond, T.S., Wiebe, D.J. (2010). Neighborhoods, daily activities, and measuring health risks experienced in urban environments. *Soc. Sci. Med.*, 71, 1943–1950. doi: 10.1016/j.socscimed.2010.09.008.

Bell, S.L., Phoenix, C., Lovell, R., Wheeler, B.W. (2015). Using GPS and geo-narratives: A methodological approach for understanding and situating everyday green space encounters: Using GPS and geo-narratives. *Area*, 47, 88–96. doi: 10.1111/area.12152.

Berkowitz, R.L., Gao, X., Michaels, E.K., Mujahid, M.S. (2020). Structurally vulnerable neighbourhood environments and racial/ethnic COVID-19 inequities. *Cities Health*, 1–4. doi: 10.1080/23748834.2020.1792069.

Bernard, P., Charafeddine, R., Frohlich, K.L., Daniel, M., Kestens, Y., Potvin, L. (2007). Health inequalities and place: A theoretical conception of neighbourhood. *Soc. Sci. Med.*, 65, 1839–1852. doi: 10.1016/j.socscimed.2007.05.037.

Braveman, P. (2006). Health disparities and health equity: Concepts and measurement. *Annu. Rev. Public Health*, 27, 167–194. doi: 10.1146/annurev.publhealth.27.021405.102103.

Browne-Yung, K., Ziersch, A., Baum, F. (2013). "Faking til you make it": Social capital accumulation of individuals on low incomes living in contrasting socio-economic neighbourhoods and its implications for health and wellbeing. *Soc. Sci. Med.*, 85, 9–17. doi: 10.1016/j.socscimed.2013.02.026.

Burgoine, T., Forouhi, N.G., Griffin, S.J., Brage, S., Wareham, N.J., Monsivais, P., (2016). Does neighborhood fast-food outlet exposure amplify inequalities in diet and obesity? A cross-sectional study. *Am. J. Clin. Nutr.*, 103, 1540–1547. doi: 10.3945/ajcn.115.128132.

Camarero, L.A. and Oliva, J. (2008). Exploring the social face of urban mobility: Daily mobility as part of the social structure in Spain. *Int. J. Urban Reg. Res.*, 32, 344–362. doi: 10.1111/j.1468-2427.2008.00778.x.

Canadian Institute for Health Information (2011). *Urban Physical Environments and Health Inequalities*. CIHI, Ottawa.

Caryl, F., Shortt, N.K., Pearce, J., Reid, G., Mitchell, R. (2020). Socioeconomic inequalities in children's exposure to tobacco retailing based on individual-level GPS data in Scotland. *Tob. Control*, 29, 367–373. doi: 10.1136/tobaccocontrol-2018-054891.

Casas, I. (2007). Social exclusion and the disabled: An accessibility approach. *Prof. Geogr.*, 59, 463–477.

Cass, N., Shove, E., Urry, J. (2005). Social exclusion, mobility and access. *Sociol. Rev.*, 53, 539–555.

Chaix, B., Merlo, J., Evans, D., Leal, C., Havard, S. (2009). Neighbourhoods in eco-epidemiologic research: Delimiting personal exposure areas. A response to Riva, Gauvin, Apparicio and Brodeur. *Soc. Sci. Med.*, 69, 1306–1310. doi: 10.1016/j.socscimed.2009.07.018.

Chaix, B., Meline, J., Duncan, S., Jardinier, L., Perchoux, C., Vallée, J., Merrien, C., Karusisi, N., Lewin, A., Brondeel, R. et al. (2013). Neighborhood environments, mobility, and health: Towards a new generation of studies in environmental health research. *Rev. Epidemiol. Santé Publique*, 61(3), S139–145. doi: 10.1016/j.respe.2013.05.017.

Chang, S., Pierson, E., Koh, P.W., Gerardin, J., Redbird, B., Grusky, D., Leskovec, J. (2020). Mobility network models of COVID-19 explain inequities and inform reopening. *Nature*. doi: 10.1038/s41586-020-2923-3.

Christian, W.J. (2012). Using geospatial technologies to explore activity-based retail food environments. *Spat. Spatiotemporal. Epidemiol.*, 3. doi: 10.1016/j.sste.2012.09.001.

Clary, C.M., Ramos, Y., Shareck, M., Kestens, Y. (2015). Should we use absolute or relative measures when assessing foodscape exposure in relation to fruit and vegetable intake? Evidence from a wide-scale Canadian study. *Prev. Med.*, 71, 83–87. doi: 10.1016/j.ypmed.2014.11.023.

Cummins, S. (2007). Commentary: Investigating neighbourhood effects on health – Avoiding the "Local Trap". *Int. J. Epidemiol.*, 36, 355–357. doi: 10.1093/ije/dym033.

Cummins, S., Curtis, S., Diez-Roux, A.V., Macintyre, S. (2007). Understanding and representing "place" in health research: A relational approach. *Soc. Sci. Med.*, 65, 1825–1838. doi: 10.1016/j.socscimed.2007.05.036.

Doherty, S.T. (ed.) (2005). *Integrated Land-Use and Transportation Models: Behavioural Foundations.* Elsevier, Amsterdam.

van Dorn, A., Cooney, R.E., Sabin, M.L. (2020). COVID-19 exacerbating inequalities in the US. *Lancet*, 395, 1243–1244. doi: 10.1016/S0140-6736(20)30893-X.

Delbosc, A. and Currie, G. (2011). The spatial context of transport disadvantage, social exclusion and well-being. *J. Transp. Geogr.*, 19, 1130–1137. doi: 10.1016/j.jtrangeo.2011.04.005.

Ella, G.A. (2020). Gender, mobility, and Covid-19: The case of Belgium. *Fem. Econ.*, 1–15. doi: 10.1080/13545701.2020.1832240.

Flamm, M. and Kaufmann, V. (2006). Operationalising the concept of motility: A qualitative study. *Mobilities*, 1, 167–189. doi: 10.1080/17450100600726563.

Frandberg, L. and Vilhelmson, B. (2011). More or less travel: Personal mobility trends in the Swedish population focusing gender and cohort. *J. Transp. Geogr.*, 19, 1235–1244. doi: 10.1016/J.Jtrangeo.2011.06.004.

Freisthler, B., Kepple, N.J., Wolf, J.P., Carson, L. (2019). Activity spaces: Assessing differences in alcohol exposures and alcohol use for parents. *GeoJournal*. doi: 10.1007/s10708-019-10059-5.

Frohlich, K.L. and De Koninck, M. (2008). *Les inégalités sociales de santé au Québec, Paramètres*. Presses de l'Université de Montréal, Montreal.

Frohlich, K.L., Mykhalovskiy, E., Miller, F., Daniel, M. (2004). Advancing the population health agenda: Encouraging the integration of social theory into population health research and practice. *Can. J. Public Health*, 95, 392–395.

Fuller, D., Gauvin, L., Kestens, Y. (2013). Individual- and area-level disparities in access to the road network, subway system and a public bicycle share program on the Island of Montreal, Canada. *Ann. Behav. Med.*, 45, 1, S95–100. doi: 10.1007/s12160-012-9433-y.

Gatrell, A.C. (2002). *Geographies of Health: An Introduction.* Blackwell, Oxford.

Giddens, A. (1984). *The Constitution of Society: Outline of the Theory of Structuration.* Polity Press, Cambridge.

Golledge, R.G. and Stimson, R.J. (1997). *Spatial Behavior: A Geographic Perspective.* Guilford Press, New York.

Gough, K.V. (2008). "Moving around": The social and spatial mobility of youth in Lusaka. *Geogr. Ann. Ser. B-Hum. Geogr.*, 90B, 243–255.

Government of Canada (2020a). The contribution of immigrants and population groups designated as visible minorities to nurse aide, orderly and patient service associate occupations [Online]. Available at: https://www150.statcan.gc.ca/n1/pub/45-28-0001/2020001/article/00036-eng.htm [Accessed 2 September 2021].

Government of Canada (2020b). COVID-19 mortality rates in Canada's ethno-cultural neighbourhoods [Online]. Available at: https://www150.statcan.gc.ca/n1/pub/45-28-0001/2020001/article/00079-eng.htm [Accessed 2 September 2021].

Hägerstrand, T. (1970). What about people in Regional Science? *Pap. Reg. Sci.*, 24, 6–21. doi: 10.1007/BF01936872.

Harvey, D. (1973). *Social Justice and the City.* E. Arnold, London.

Hawkes, S. and Buse, K. (2020). COVID-19 and the gendered markets of people and products: Explaining inequalities in infections and deaths. *Can. J. Dev. Stud. Rev. Can. Détudes Dév.*, 1–18. doi: 10.1080/02255189.2020.1824894.

Inagami, S., Cohen, D.A., Finch, B.K. (2007). Non-residential neighborhood exposures suppress neighborhood effects on self-rated health. *Soc. Sci. Med.*, 65, 1779–1791. doi: 10.1016/j.socscimed.2007.05.051.

Jiron, P. (2007). Unravelling invisible inequalities in the city through urban daily mobility. The Case of Santiago de Chile. *Swiss J. Sociol.*, 33, 45–68.

Kaufmann, V. (2011). *Rethinking the City: Urban Dynamics and Motility*, 1st edition. Routledge, Oxford.

Kaufmann, V., Bergman, M.M., Joye, D. (2004). Motility: Mobility as capital. *Int. J. Urban Reg. Res.*, 28, 745–756. doi: 10.1111/j.0309-1317.2004.00549.x.

Kaufmann, V., Dubois, Y., Ravalet, E. (2018). Measuring and typifying mobility using motility. *Appl. Mobilities*, 3, 198–213. doi: 10.1080/23800127.2017.1364540.

Kawachi, I. and Berkman, L.F. (eds) (2003). *Neighborhoods and Health.* Oxford University Press, New York.

Kestens, Y., Lebel, A., Daniel, M., Thériault, M., Pampalon, R. (2010). Using experienced activity spaces to measure foodscape exposure. *Health Place*, 16. doi: 10.1016/j.healthplace.2010.06.016.

Kestens, Y., Lebel, A., Chaix, B., Clary, C., Daniel, M., Pampalon, R., Theriault, M., Subramanian, S.V. (2012). Association between activity space exposure to food establishments and individual risk of overweight. *PLoS ONE*, 7, e41418. doi: 10.1371/journal.pone.0041418.

Kim, J. and Kwan, M.-P. (2021). How neighborhood effect averaging might affect assessment of individual exposures to air pollution: A study of ozone exposures in Los Angeles. *Ann. Am. Assoc. Geogr.*, 111, 121–140. doi: 10.1080/24694452.2020.1756208.

Kimbro, R.T., Sharp, G., Denney, J.T. (2017). Home and away: Area socioeconomic disadvantage and obesity risk. *Health Place*, 44, 94–102. doi: 10.1016/j.healthplace.2017.02.001.

Kirchner, T.R., Cantrell, J., Anesetti-Rothermel, A., Ganz, O., Vallone, D.M., Abrams, D.B. (2013). Geospatial exposure to point-of-sale tobacco: Real-time craving and smoking-cessation outcomes. *Am. J. Prev. Med.*, 45, 379–385.

Krivo, L.J., Washington, H.M., Peterson, R.D., Browning, C.R., Calder, C.A., Kwan, M.P. (2013). Social isolation of disadvantage and advantage: The reproduction of inequality in urban space. *Soc. Forces*, 92, 141–164. doi: 10.1093/sf/sot043.

Kwan, M.P. (2000). Gender differences in space-time constraints. *Area*, 32, 145–156.

Kwan, M.P. (2009). From place-based to people-based exposure measures. *Soc. Sci. Med.*, 69, 1311–1313. doi: 10.1016/j.socscimed.2009.07.013.

Lebel, A., Kestens, Y., Pampalon, R., Theriault, M., Daniel, M., Subramanian, S.V. (2012). Local context influence, activity space, and foodscape exposure in two Canadian metropolitan settings: Is daily mobility exposure associated with overweight? *J. Obes.*, 912645. doi: 10.1155/2012/912645.

Lipperman-Kreda, S., Morrison, C., Grube, J.W., Gaidus, A. (2015). Youth activity spaces and daily exposure to tobacco outlets. *Health Place*, 34, 30–33. doi: 10.1016/j.healthplace.2015.03.013.

Manderscheid, K. (2009). Integrating space and mobilities into the analysis of social inequality. *Distinktion Scand. J. Soc. Theory*, 10, 7–27. doi: 10.1080/1600910x.2009.9672739.

Manderscheid, K. (2014). Criticising the solitary mobile subject: Researching relational mobilities and reflecting on mobile methods. *Mobilities*, 9, 188–219. doi: 10.1080/17450101.2013.830406.

Marmot, M., Allen, J., Boyce, T., Goldblatt, P., Morrison, J. (2020a). Health equity in England: The Marmot review 10 years on – Executive summary. Report, Institute of Health Equity, London.

Marmot, M., Allen, J., Goldblatt, P., Herd, E., Morrison, J. (2020b). Build back fairer: The COVID-19 Marmot review. The pandemic, socioeconomic and health inequalities in England. Report, Institute of Health Equity, London.

Mason, M.J. and Korpela, K. (2009). Activity spaces and urban adolescent substance use and emotional health. *J. Adolesc.*, 32, 925–939. doi: 10.1016/j.adolescence.2008.08.004.

Matthews, S.A., Detwiler, J.E., Burton, L.M. (2005). Geo-ethnography: Coupling geographic information analysis techniques with ethnographic methods in urban research. *Cartogr. Int. J. Geogr. Inf. Geovisualization*, 40, 75–90. doi: 10.3138/2288-1450-W061-R664.

McPherson, M., Smith-Lovin, L., Cook, J.M. (2001). Birds of a feather: Homophily in social networks. *Annu. Rev. Sociol.*, 27, 415–444. doi: 10.1146/annurev.soc.27.1.415.

Miciukiewicz, K. and Vigar, G. (2012). Mobility and social cohesion in the splintered city: Challenging technocentric transport research and policy-making practices. *Urban Stud.*, 49, 1941–1957. doi: 10.1177/0042098012444886.

Mitra, R., Moore, S.A., Gillespie, M., Faulkner, G., Vanderloo, L.M., Chulak-Bozzer, T., Rhodes, R.E., Brussoni, M., Tremblay, M.S. (2020). Healthy movement behaviours in children and youth during the COVID-19 pandemic: Exploring the role of the neighbourhood environment. *Health Place*, 65, 102418. doi: 10.1016/j.healthplace.2020.102418.

Morency, C., Paez, A., Roorda, M.J., Mercado, R., Farber, S. (2011). Distance traveled in three Canadian cities: Spatial analysis from the perspective of vulnerable population segments. *J. Transp. Geogr.*, 19, 39–50. doi: 10.1016/j.jtrangeo.2009.09.013.

Morrison, C.N., Byrnes, H.F., Miller, B.A., Kaner, E., Wiehe, S.E., Ponicki, W.R., Wiebe, D.J. (2019). Assessing individuals' exposure to environmental conditions using residence-based measures, activity location-based measures, and activity path-based measures. *Epidemiology*, 30, 166–176. doi: 10.1097/EDE.0000000000000940.

Naess, P. (2006). Accessibility, activity participation and location of activities: Exploring the links between residential location and travel behaviour. *Urban Stud.*, 43, 627–652.

Paez, A., Gertes Mercado, R., Farber, S., Morency, C., Roorda, M. (2010). Relative accessibility deprivation indicators for urban settings: Definitions and application to food deserts in Montreal. *Urban Stud.*, 47, 1415–1438. doi: 10.1177/0042098009353626.

Perchoux, C., Chaix, B., Brondeel, R., Kestens, Y. (2016). Residential buffer, perceived neighborhood, and individual activity space: New refinements in the definition of exposure areas – The RECORD cohort study. *Health Place*, 40, 116–122. doi: 10.1016/j.healthplace.2016.05.004.

Poland, B., Frohlich, K., Haines, R.J., Mykhalovskiy, E., Rock, M., Sparks, R. (2006). The social context of smoking: The next frontier in tobacco control? *Tob. Control*, 15, 59–63. doi: 10.1136/tc.2004.009886.

Pred, A. (1977). The choreography of existence: Comments on Hägerstrand's time-geography and its usefulness. *Econ. Geogr.*, 53, 207–221.

Preston, J. and Rajé, F. (2007). Accessibility, mobility and transport-related social exclusion. *J. Transp. Geogr.*, 15, 151–160. doi: 10.1016/j.jtrangeo.2006.05.002.

Public Health Ontario (2020). COVID-19 in Ontario – A focus on diversity: January 15 2020 to May 14 2020. Report, Queen's Printer for Ontario, Toronto.

Ramadier, T., Lee-Gosselin, M.E.H., Frenette, A. (2005). Conceptual perspectives for explaining spatio-temporal behaviour in urban areas. In *Integrated Land-Use and Transportation Models*, Lee-Gosselin, M.E.H. and Doherty, S.T. (eds). Emerald Group Publishing Limited, Leeds.

Reynolds, T. (2013). "Them and us": "Black neighbourhoods" as a social capital resource among black youths living in inner-city London. *Urban Stud.*, 50, 484–498. doi: 10.1177/0042098012468892.

Ritchie, H., Mathieu, E., Rodés-Guirao, L., Appel, C., Giattino, C., Ortiz-Ospina, E., Hasell, J., Macdonald, B., Beltekian, D., Roser, M. (2020). Coronavirus pandemic (COVID-19): Stay-at-home restrictions. Report, Our World in Data, Oxford.

Riva, M., Gauvin, L., Barnett, T.A. (2007). Toward the next generation of research into small area effects on health: A synthesis of multilevel investigations published since July 1998. *J. Epidemiol. Community Health*, 61, 853–861. doi: 10.1136/jech.2006.050740.

Rodriguez, D.A., Cho, G.H., Evenson, K.R., Conway, T.L., Cohen, D., Ghosh-Dastidar, B., Pickrel, J.L., Veblen-Mortenson, S., Lytle, L.A. (2012). Out and about: Association of the built environment with physical activity behaviors of adolescent females. *Health Place*, 18, 55–62. doi: 10.1016/j.healthplace.2011.08.020.

Schönfelder, S. and Axhausen, K.W. (2003). Activity spaces: Measures of social exclusion? *Transp. Policy*, 10, 273–286. doi: 10.1016/j.tranpol.2003.07.002.

Sen, A. (1999). *Development as Freedom*. Random Books, New York.

Shareck, M., Frohlich, K.L., Kestens, Y. (2014a). Considering daily mobility for a more comprehensive understanding of contextual effects on social inequalities in health: A conceptual proposal. *Health Place*, 29, 154–160. doi: 10.1016/j.healthplace.2014.07.007.

Shareck, M., Kestens, Y., Frohlich, K.L. (2014b). Moving beyond the residential neighborhood to explore social inequalities in exposure to area-level disadvantage: Results from the Interdisciplinary Study on Inequalities in Smoking. *Soc. Sci. Med.*, 1982, 108, 106–114. doi: 10.1016/j.socscimed.2014.02.044.

Shareck, M., Kestens, Y., Vallée, J., Datta, G., Frohlich, K.L. (2015). The added value of accounting for activity space when examining the association between tobacco retailer availability and smoking among young adults. *Tob. Control*. doi: 10.1136/tobaccocontrol-2014-052194.

Shareck, M., Datta, G.D., Vallée, J., Kestens, Y., Frohlich, K.L. (2018a). Is smoking cessation in young adults associated with tobacco retailer availability in their activity space? *Nicotine & Tobacco Research.* doi: 10.1093/ntr/nty242.

Shareck, M., Lewis, D., Smith, N.R., Clary, C., Cummins, S. (2018b). Associations between home and school neighbourhood food environments and adolescents' fast-food and sugar-sweetened beverage intakes: Findings from the Olympic Regeneration in East London (ORiEL) Study. *Public Health Nutr.*, 21, 2842–2851. doi: 10.1017/S1368980018001477.

Sharp, G. and Kimbro, R.T. (2021). Neighborhood social environments, healthy resources, and adult diabetes: Accounting for activity space exposures. *Health Place*, 67, 102473. doi: 10.1016/j.healthplace.2020.102473.

Sharp, G., Denney, J.T., Kimbro, R.T. (2015). Multiple contexts of exposure: Activity spaces, residential neighborhoods, and self-rated health. *Soc. Sci. Med.*, 146, 204–213. doi: 10.1016/j.socscimed.2015.10.040.

Sheller, M. and Urry, J. (2006). The new mobilities paradigm. *Environ. Plan.*, A38, 207–226.

Shin, H. (2011). Spatial capability for understanding gendered mobility for Korean Christian immigrant women in Los Angeles. *Urban Stud.*, 48, 2355–2373 [Online]. Available at: https://doi.org/10.1177/0042098010388955.

Shortt, N.K., Tisch, C., Pearce, J., Richardson, E.A., Mitchell, R. (2014). The density of tobacco retailers in home and school environments and relationship with adolescent smoking behaviours in Scotland. *Tob. Control.* doi: 10.1136/tobaccocontrol-2013-051473.

Skelton, T. (2013). Young people's urban im/mobilities: Relationality and identity formation. *Urban Stud.*, 50, 467–483. doi: 10.1177/0042098012468893.

Soja, E.W. (2010). *Seeking Spatial Justice.* University of Minnesota Press, Minneapolis.

Spinney, J.E.L., Scott, D.M., Newbold, K.B. (2009). Transport mobility benefits and qua-lity of life: A time-use perspective of elderly Canadians. *Transp. Policy*, 16, 1–11. doi: 10.1016/j.tranpol.2009.01.002.

Stanley, J.K., Hensher, D.A., Stanley, J.R., Vella-Brodrick, D. (2011). Mobility, social exclusion and well-being: Exploring the links. *Transp. Res. Part Policy Pract.*, 45, 789–801. doi: 10.1016/j.tra.2011.06.007.

Urry, J. (2007). *Mobilities.* Polity, Cambridge.

Vallée, J., Cadot, E., Grillo, F., Parizot, I., Chauvin, P. (2010). The combined effects of activity space and neighbourhood of residence on participation in preventive healthcare activities: The case of cervical screening in the Paris metropolitan area (France). *Health Place*, 16, 838–852. doi: 10.1016/j.healthplace.2010.04.009.

Vallée, J., Cadot, E., Roustit, C., Parizot, I., Chauvin, P. (2011). The role of daily mobility in mental health inequalities: The interactive influence of activity space and neighbourhood of residence on depression. *Soc. Sci. Med.*, 73, 1133–1144. doi: 10.1016/j.socscimed.2011.08.009.

Weill, J.A., Stigler, M., Deschenes, O., Springborn, M.R. (2020). Social distancing responses to COVID-19 emergency declarations strongly differentiated by income. *Proc. Natl. Acad. Sci.*, 117, 19658–19660. doi: 10.1073/pnas.2009412117.

Weiss, A. (2005). The transnationalization of social inequality: Conceptualizing social positions on a world scale. *Curr. Sociol.*, 53, 707–728. doi: 10.1177/0011392105052722.

White, R.J. and Green, A.E. (2011). Opening up or closing down opportunities? The role of social networks and attachment to place in informing young peoples' attitudes and access to training and employment. *Urban Stud.*, 48, 41–60. doi: 10.1177/0042098009360234.

Woolf, S.H., Masters, R.K., Aron, L.Y. (2021). Effect of the Covid-19 pandemic in 2020 on life expectancy across populations in the USA and other high income countries: Simulations of provisional mortality data. *BMJ*, 373, n1343. doi: 10.1136/bmj.n1343.

World Health Organization (2008). Commission des déterminants sociaux de la santé. Combler le fossé dans une génération. Instaurer l'équité en santé en agissant sur les déterminants sociaux de la santé. Meeting Report.

Zenk, S.N., Schulz, A.J., Matthews, S.A., Odoms-Young, A., Wilbur, J., Wegrzyn, L., Gibbs, K., Braunschweig, C., Stokes, C. (2011). Activity space environment and dietary and physical activity behaviors: A pilot study. *Health Place*, 17, 1150–1161. doi: 10.1016/j.healthplace.2011.05.001.

Zhai, W., Liu, M., Peng, Z.-R. (2021). Social distancing and inequality in the United States amid COVID-19 outbreak. *Environ. Plan. Econ. Space*, 53, 3–5. doi: 10.1177/0308518X20932576.

# PART 2

# Everyday Environments and Active Modes of Travel

# 4

# Walking in Everyday Life: The Built Environment and Pedestrian Insecurity

**Marie-Soleil CLOUTIER and Karine LACHAPELLE**
*LAPS, Institut national de la recherche scientifique, Montreal, Canada*

Walking is the very essence of biped human beings, one of the first accomplishments we expect of our infants and the last thing we let go of as we age (Arason 2014). Nevertheless, walking has too often been underestimated in daily chains of movement, despite its representing both a source of physical activity and the easiest means of transport to cover short distances. In fact, the physical and mental health benefits of walking have long been well documented in the scientific literature, including lower rates of chronic conditions such as obesity and cardiovascular disease as well as benefits for depression, by encouraging social interaction (Lee and Buchner 2008; Guo and Gandavarapu 2010; Mammen and Faulkner 2013).

This chapter has four complementary goals. First, we will briefly review the five dimensions characterizing walkability in the urban environment, based on recent works on the subject (section 4.1). Secondly (sections 4.2 and 4.3), we will present the different sources of pedestrian insecurity, in particular the risk pedestrians incur in relation to road traffic and its most well-known influencing factors. Section 4.4 will be dedicated to two interventions (Vision Zero and speed reduction) aimed at enhancing

---

For a color version of all the figures in this chapter, see www.iste.co.uk/vallee/everyday.zip.

*Everyday Mobility and Health*,

pedestrian safety. Finally, this chapter concludes (section 4.5) with two avenues of research that require greater attention from the scientific community and the actors in the field: accurate measurements of pedestrian exposure and the evaluation of interventions.

## 4.1. The dimensions of walkability

Walkability is officially defined as the "degree of safety, aesthetic and interest of a pedestrian route" (Quebec Board of the French Language 2009). This is how a "pedestrian-friendly" environment – adapted to the pedestrian's scale and needs – encourages the practice of walking not only for moving from one place to another, but also for socializing and leisure purposes. In concrete terms, at a local scale, walkability is measurable by a set of criteria that can be observed in the environment (Raulin et al. 2016; Dovey and Pafka 2020). This chapter focuses on urban spaces because utilitarian walking is more frequent there than in rural spaces. However, rural spaces are not exempt from walkability concerns: some of our observations based on urban studies can also be transposed to rural roads.

The existence of a link between the urban form and citizens' modal choices is at the heart of research on walkability. Cervero and Kockelman (1997) were the first to discuss this link in an article in which they assert that the demand for transport is intrinsically related to the three dimensions of urban form: design, density and diversity, also called the 3 "Ds". More recently, several authors have suggested adding two other "Ds": destination accessibility and distance to public transport networks (Ewing and Cervero 2010). Furthermore, some authors working on active mobility (including walking), argue that the elements from the natural and the built environment related to the quality of the walking experience and pedestrian comfort are also important features to add to this conceptualization of the link between urban form and transport (Cerin et al. 2006; Clifton et al. 2007; Chaudhury et al. 2011; Lee and Talen 2014; Negron-Poblete and Lord 2014; Paquin 2015; Khanal and Mateo-Babiano 2016; Moura et al. 2017; Lee and Dean 2018; Al Shammas and Escobar 2019; Mukhtar et al. 2019). Here, we will consider some of these additions to explore walkability across five dimensions: not only those highlighted by Cervero and Kockelman (design, density, diversity), but also those related to destinations and the quality and comfort of pedestrians (Figure 4.1). The following sections will explore these dimensions in detail.

### 4.1.1. *Design*

Design here refers to the elements of the road network, the true skeleton of our post-industrial cities, as well as the physical or natural barriers found on pedestrian routes.

One of the most common indicators mentioned in the walkability literature is the sidewalk (presence, width, slope, quality of materials, maintenance including snow removal, temporary or permanent obstruction, etc.) (Clifton et al. 2007; Chaudhury et al. 2011; Lee and Talen 2014; Negron-Poblete and Lord 2014; Paquin 2015; Moura et al. 2017; Lee and Dean 2018). Special attention has been given to sidewalk continuity along the street sections and connectivity within or outside the street network, essential features for quality walks (Clifton et al. 2007; Paquin 2015; Moura et al. 2017).

Road network connectivity – regardless of the presence of a sidewalk – is also mentioned in various walkability indices (Khanal and Mateo-Babiano 2016). Other characteristics of the road network such as road width, vehicle number or speed limits are also important due to their influence on the pedestrian experience (Clifton et al. 2007; Chaudhury et al. 2011; Maghelal and Capp 2011; Lee and Talen 2014; Negron-Poblete and Lord 2014; Paquin 2015; Mukhtar et al. 2019).

The intersection, an obligatory passage for pedestrians in any urban setting, is also taken into account in many walkability indices. That includes elements to help pedestrians cross safely: pedestrian crossings (presence, width, visibility, etc.) or proper signaling (stop signs, traffic lights and pedestrian lights) (Clifton et al. 2007; Chaudhury et al. 2011; Lee and Talen 2014; Negron-Poblete and Lord 2014; Paquin 2015; Lee and Dean 2018).

Finally, streams, rivers, ditches, highways or power lines not only create physical barriers but sometimes also psychological barriers to walking within and between neighborhoods. However, these seem not to be taken into account in the walkability indices surveyed, with a few exceptions (Clifton et al. 2007; Lee and Talen 2014).

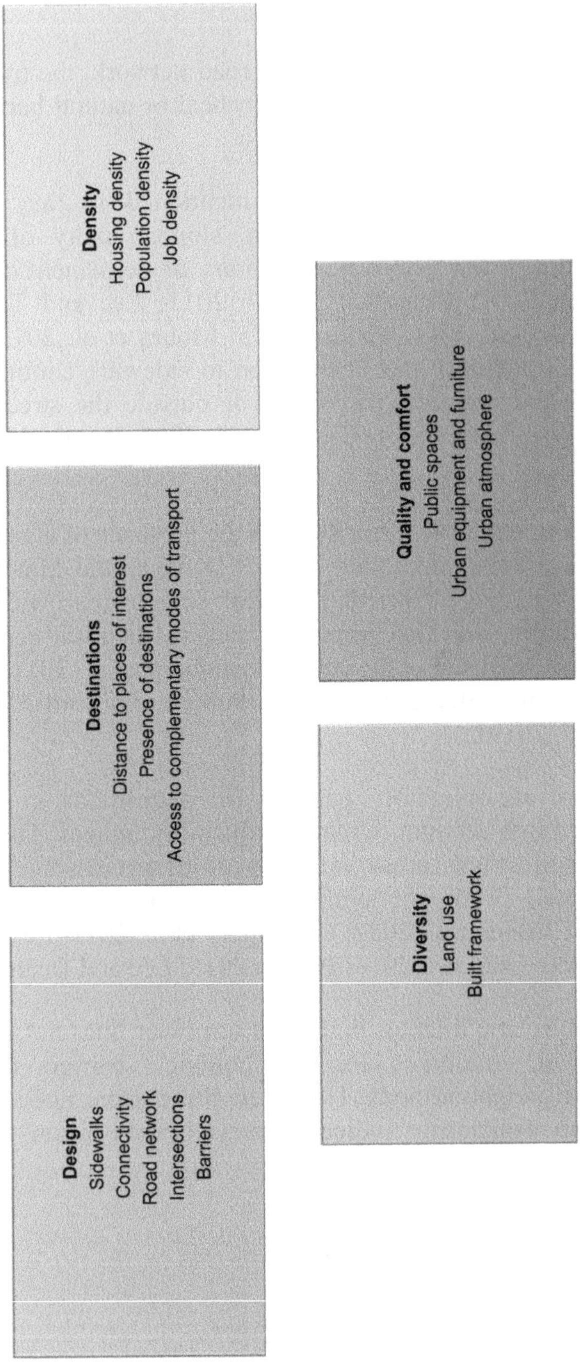


**Figure 4.1.** *Walkability dimensions and main indicators*

### 4.1.2. *Destinations*

The "destinations" dimension refers to the amount and proximity of places people can reach on foot as potential destinations: it has been recognized that the proximity of places of interest (measured in time/minutes or distance/meters) promotes walking.

This dimension includes three subgroups of indicators:

– the distances between the origin and destination (O–D), which provide information on the spatial dispersion of journeys and on the feasibility of reaching those destinations on foot (Frank et al. 2005, 2010; Adams et al. 2014; Vale et al. 2016);

– the presence of interesting destinations, including (public and private) services (such as parks, community centers, libraries) and essential shops, as well as schools, hospitals, grocery stores, pharmacies, etc. (Lee and Talen 2014; Mukhtar et al. 2019; Saghapur et al. 2019);

– access to complementary modes of transport (public transport, cycling network, self-service bicycle station), to reach further destinations and incorporating walking as part of the travel chain (Cerin et al. 2006; Vargo et al. 2012; Negron-Poblete and Lord 2014; Lee and Dean 2018; Mukhtar et al. 2019).

### 4.1.3. *Density*

The "density" dimension concerns compact and populated urban forms that facilitate the adoption of walking. Three types of density are commonly used for calculating walkability indices and identifying population pools likely to choose walking as a mode of transport from their places of residence or workplaces: housing density, population density (residents) and employment density (Cerin et al. 2006; Frank et al. 2010; Maghelal and Capp 2011; Vargo et al. 2012; Adams et al. 2014; Giles-Corti et al. 2014; Lee and Talen 2014; Khanal and Mateo-Babiano 2016; Vale et al. 2016; Stockton et al. 2016; Al Shammas and Escobar 2019; Mukhtar et al. 2019). These indicators complement those previously mentioned relating to destinations.

### 4.1.4. *Diversity*

The diversity dimension is based on the connection between diverse environments and a pedestrian-friendly experience. It involves focusing on the type of buildings and the built environment (Clifton et al. 2007; Chaudhury et al. 2011; Maghelal and Capp 2011) as well as on land use. The diversity dimension is almost systematically used in walkability indices because it reveals a territory's diversity based on its uses and its zoning (commercial, residential, industrial, etc.), also known as functional mix, without counting any specific places as in the destinations dimension (Clifton et al. 2007; Chaudhury et al. 2011; Maghelal and Capp 2011; Adams et al. 2014; Giles-Corti et al. 2014; Lee and Talen 2014; Negron-Poblete and Lord 2014; Paquin 2015; Khanal and Mateo-Babiano 2016; Moura et al. 2017; Lee and Dean 2018; Al Shammas and Escobar 2019; Mukhtar et al. 2019).

### 4.1.5. *Quality and comfort*

The pedestrian "quality and comfort" dimension extends the indicators relating to the "design" dimension and focuses on routes at a local scale. Some of these elements are subjective in nature since the comfort and quality of a journey may vary depending on the walker. The presence of public spaces and amenities such as lighting and benches (including their upkeep) is of the utmost importance, not to mention the presence of trees and vegetation to grant shade and freshness (Clifton et al. 2007; Chaudhury et al. 2011; Maghelal and Capp 2011; Lee and Talen 2014; Negron-Poblete and Lord 2014; Paquin 2015; Lee and Dean 2018; Al Shammas and Escobar 2019). Other "service points" are also mentioned in some works: rain shelters, garbage cans, post boxes, toilets and water fountains (Clifton et al. 2007; Maghelal and Capp 2011; Lord and Negron-Poblete 2014; Paquin 2015).

A second subgroup of elements falling under the "quality and comfort" dimension relates to the urban atmosphere and architectural richness along the walking routes. These characteristics can influence the perceptions of city dwellers and their decision to walk or not. For example, some authors use an aesthetic indicator that includes aspects such as incivility (graffiti, cleanliness), gardening and the presence of attractions (Clifton et al. 2007; Chaudhury et al. 2011; Lee and Talen 2014; Negron-Poblete and Lord 2014; Paquin 2015; Vale et al. 2016; Lee and Dean 2018; Al Shammas and

Escobar 2019). Other studies also point to building and soil maintenance as qualitative indicators of a good atmosphere (Clifton et al. 2007; Chaudhury et al. 2011; Negron-Poblete and Lord 2014; Paquin 2015; Lee and Dean 2018). Facade transparency or architectural variety and visual cues in space are all elements that contribute to the urban atmosphere (Lee and Talen 2014; Negron-Poblete and Lord 2014; Moura et al. 2017). Despite rarely being mentioned in the literature (Maghelal and Capp 2011; Al Shammas and Escobar 2019), air pollution and noise have an impact on the pedestrian experience. However, they are difficult to measure and this may explain why they are not often integrated into walkability indices.

This chapter provides a general picture of the elements found in the five dimensions of walkability indices. Let us insist on the fact that these elements are based on various data and different geographical scales. At a local scale, walkability is assessed by means of the built environment, which involves collecting data in situ (Maghelal and Capp 2011). These field-related qualitative measures also encompass the quality and comfort dimension, as well as certain design criteria. At a larger scale, walkability is measured systematically with geographical data available on the entire territory studied (Saelens et al. 2003). Such quantitative measures usually provide more information on the diversity, density and destination dimensions, as well as measurable criteria on design.

Regardless of the data and scales used for creating walkability indices, we should emphasize that dimensions are generally considered as a whole, variables being interdependent, which makes it difficult to disentangle their respective influence. It is for this reason that most walkability indices introduce different weights for each of the variables considered, or even combine them differently depending on the subsequent uses of the index. For example, a walkability index designed for older populations places more emphasis on essential variables for senior walkers, such as the presence of benches, sidewalks or traffic lights at intersections (Huguenin-Richard and Cloutier 2021) – for further information on the heterogeneity of environmental effects on walking, see Chapter 5.

## 4.2. The experience of insecurity: when walking is a source of fear

Pedestrian safety is a cross-cutting element that engages almost every dimension of walkability (the design of streets and intersections, the accessibility and diversity of destinations or the quality and comfort of walkways). This can involve fear of the other (as in the fear of being attacked, especially among women) or fear of oneself (the fear of falling on public roads, especially among the elderly). Both of these fears need to be addressed since they can affect day-to-day mobility through the modal choices they give rise to.

### 4.2.1. *Personal safety and walking: fear of the other among women*

One of the dominant themes in research on women walking is the perception of insecurity (criminality) and in particular, the fear of being attacked in places regarded as dangerous, often due to inadequate urban planning that neglects pedestrian needs (Valentine 1989; Paquin 2002; Clifton and Livi 2005). Along the same lines, Fenster (2005) argues that what prevents women from exercising their right to the city is the fear of using public spaces – especially the street, public transport and urban parks – due to the fear of the other. Vaughn (2011) states that the sense of insecurity is a deterrent to walking and cycling as a means of transport: women voluntarily restrict their mobility because they are more sensitive to the feeling of safety in these modes of transport. Note that some works on walkability address this type of insecurity by including police records (number of assaults and burglaries, enforcement of pedestrian regulations, etc.) or observations on the urban atmosphere (the fact of being seen and heard) in their walkability indices (Maghelal and Capp 2011; Lee and Talen 2014; Vale et al. 2016; Moura et al. 2017). Yet, these concerns for personal safety constitute one of the blind spots of daily walking mobility because little is done by the authorities to reduce the real sources and the perceptions of danger. This could be achieved by redeveloping urban public spaces, and the street in particular.

### 4.2.2. *Walking and falling: fear of oneself among seniors*

As we age, our perception of difficulties related to walking increases, primarily in relation to walking speed, street-crossing and the fear of falling in public spaces (Huguenin-Richard et al. 2014). In Canada and Quebec, falling (including at home and outside, on public roads), is one of the leading causes of injury and hospitalization among people over 65 (Public Health Agency of Canada 2014; Gagné et al. 2018), a similar statistic to the one found in the rest of the world (World Health Organization 2018a). These falls sometimes have dramatic consequences on the autonomy and mobility of seniors, including the fear of falling again, which leads to a reduction in walking frequency. Yet, very few studies of outdoor falls examine their impact in the toll of injured pedestrians, or look into their environmental causes (Oxley et al. 2018). A review of the literature published in 2017 also suggests that victims of outdoor falls are generally in good shape, leaving the typical age-related health problems aside (Schepers et al. 2017). According to the research, victims blame poor road conditions as the cause of their fall, an estimated 40% of those injured in the Gyllencreutz et al. study. (2015).

Winter (accompanied by harsher weather conditions such as sleet or snow in several Western countries) creates a propitious setting for falling at all ages, but all the more so in people aged 65 or over. The Canadian Community Health Survey (CCHS) from 2009 to 2010 reported that 16% of people who fell were "walking on a snowy or icy surface" (Public Health Agency of Canada 2014). The study by Morency et al. (2012) conducted in December 2008 and January 2009 confirmed these statistics based on reports from ambulance interventions following a fall. In this sample, 30% of the reported falls had taken place outdoors, among which 41% involved a person aged 65 or over. In fact, slippery sidewalks and road surfaces with an accumulation of snow and/or ice increase falls (Bjornstig et al. 1997; Bélanger-Bonneau et al. 2002; Gyllencreutz et al. 2015), with the consequences this entails. A US survey reported that people over 65 are twice as likely to report having difficulty leaving the house when it is cold compared to younger people (Clarke et al. 2015). In another Vancouver study, seniors (even those who lived in neighborhoods with high walkability) decreased attendance to destinations within walking distance by 25% when there was snow (Clarke et al. 2017). The fear of falling has implications for the decision to walk, particularly in winter.

## 4.3. Road safety and walking: potential danger when crossing

In road safety terms, "risk" refers to the probability of a collision in two dimensions: the occurrence frequency and the severity of consequences (property damage, injury, death) (Hauer 1982; Haight 1986). In addition to this definition, some road users are more vulnerable than others to risk, according to three criteria: the absence of a protective "shell" in traffic to protect themselves against kinetic energy (e.g. pedestrians, cyclists and, to some extent, motorcyclists); the ability or not to perform other tasks while immersed in traffic (for instance, children and older adults); and resilience in the event of injuries (e.g. people who are aging or suffering from prior impairments) (Hakkert and Braimaister 2002). Briefly stated, pedestrians are vulnerable users for whom the risks of injury and death are uneven, due to their mode of transport.

### 4.3.1. *Global portrait of collisions involving pedestrians*

The Global Status Report on Road Safety 2018, published by the World Health Organization (WHO), indicated that 23% of road fatalities around the world involved pedestrians (Figure 4.2) (WHO 2018b). On the other hand, compared to other road users, the proportion of pedestrian fatalities varied from region to region: from 14% in Southeast Asia to 25% in developed regions such as the Americas, Europe and the Western Pacific, and up to 40% in Africa. Although these figures partly reflect the prevailing form of mobility in these regions, the burden of death or injury to pedestrians represents a significant health problem which is not without effect on the propensity of the population to adopt walking on a daily basis when other modes of transport are available.

Cities are a major contributor to the burden of pedestrian fatalities and injuries in high-income countries. For example, in the early 2010s, the proportion of accidents causing pedestrian fatalities in urban areas was 70% in the European Union and 76% in the United States (World Health Organization 2013). This is not surprising as these countries generally concentrate the most pedestrians and moving vehicles in the cities.

The most recent report from the Organization for Economic Cooperation and Development (OECD) on the subject indicates that the greatest progress in preventing fatalities has been made among motor vehicle occupants rather than pedestrians, particularly those aged 65 or over (International Transport Forum 2020). In the United States, the number of deaths in car accidents decreased by 27% between 2000 and 2009, while the decrease was only 14% for pedestrians (Transportation for America 2011). Even more alarming, the "Dangerous by Design" report revealed a 45% increase in pedestrian fatalities between 2010 and 2019 in the United States (Transportation for America 2021).

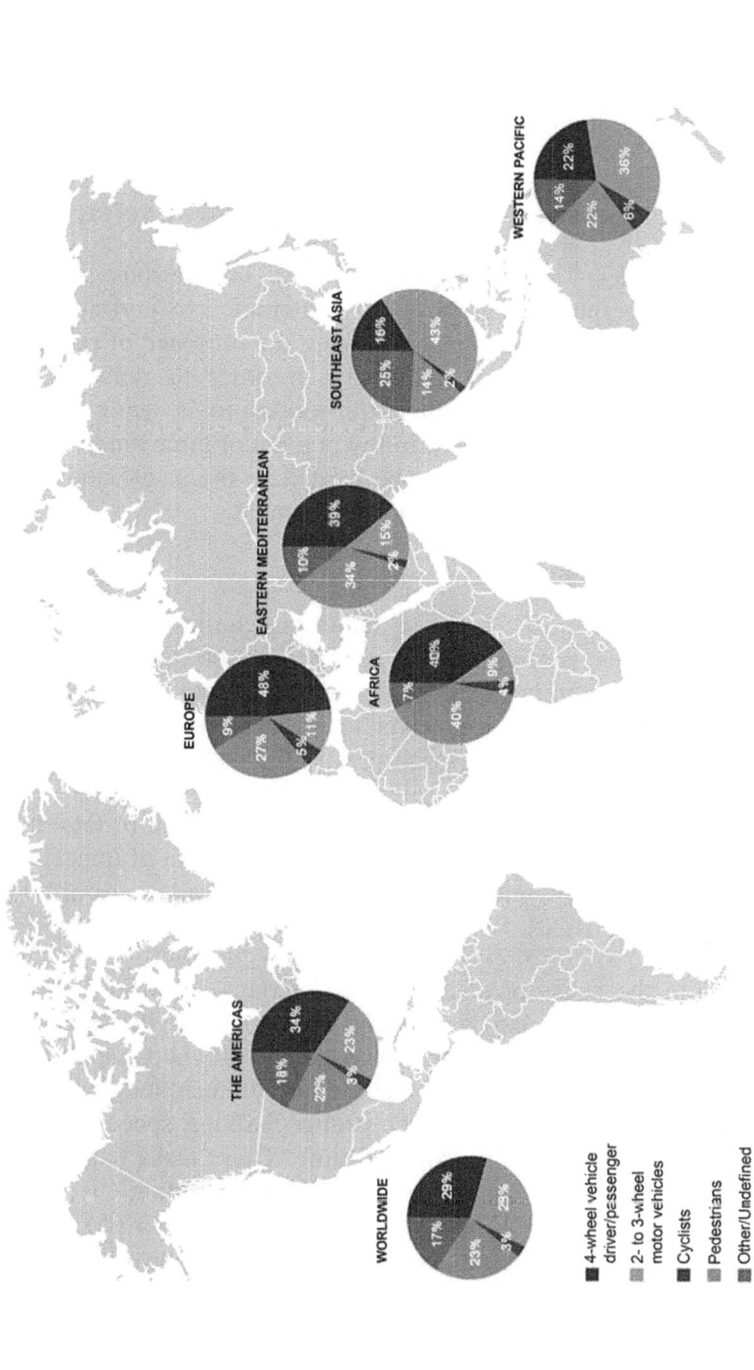


**Figure 4.2.** *Fatality distribution by type of road user in different WHO regions (source: World Health Organization 2018b)*

In low-income countries, while the burden of pedestrian injuries is high in almost all cities, it can also be high in rural[1] areas, depending on the degree of local motorization (Kobusingye et al. 2001; Ghaffar et al. 2004; Moshiro et al. 2005; Labinjo et al. 2009).

## 4.3.2. *Risk factors associated with pedestrian road safety*

In recent decades, many works drawing on various disciplines (engineering, ethnography, geography) have attempted to portray different risk factors associated with collisions involving the presence of pedestrians. The goal is to intervene more effectively in order to reduce injuries, particularly in a context where active transportation is being promoted. These factors, briefly described in the following, are of three kinds. They can take place at the level of individuals, be related to the social and political context, or involve the road and the built environment.

### 4.3.2.1. *Individual behaviors*

At the individual level, the first risk factor is determined by the driving speed of drivers: this speed has an impact both on the occurrence of collisions, as well as on injury severity during the impact. A greater driving speed implies shorter time for the driver to see and react to danger, and a longer stopping distance if a pedestrian gets in the way (see Figure 4.3(a)), thus increasing the likelihood of a collision. When these collisions are not avoided, the impact speed directly determines the likelihood of fatal injuries (see Figure 4.3(b)). Death of a pedestrian who has been hit at impact speeds of 30 km/h or less is highly unlikely, but almost certain at speeds of 80 km/h or over (Vivre en ville 2020).

In addition to the behavior of drivers, pedestrians – and in particular at crossings – must be taken into account in risk analysis. Pedestrians must perform several complex tasks when crossing a street: choosing a place and a time for crossing, making sure they can see and be seen, judging the speed of approaching cars and calculating the proper walking speed to complete the crossing before the end of the allotted time. These tasks require actions many population subgroups cannot safely perform in certain environments. For example, children under 12 and senior pedestrians (over 65) can find it difficult to perform such actions, mainly due to their physical condition

1. Solutions to pedestrian road accidents in rural areas, which are likely to be quite different due to lower densities and higher speeds, will not be addressed in this chapter.

(smaller size in children, slow walking speed in seniors) and cognitive abilities. For further details, see Tournier et al. (2016) for seniors, and Cloutier et al. (2021) for children, among others.

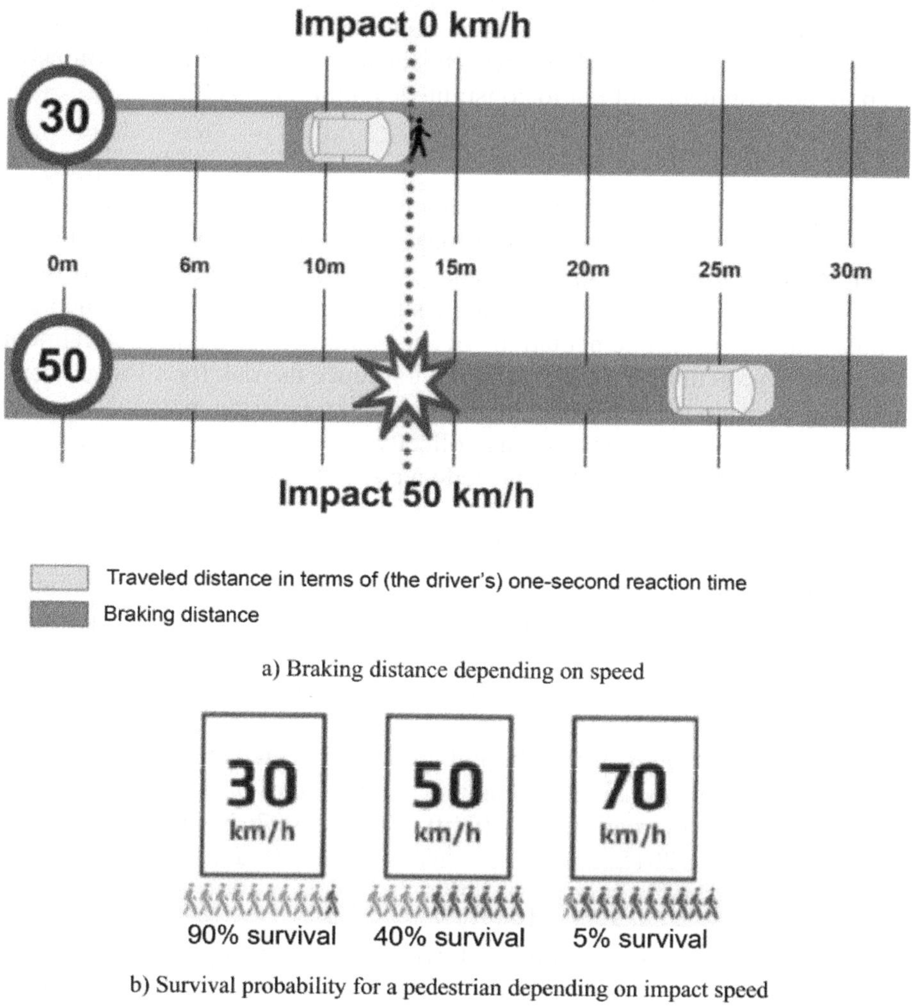


**Figure 4.3.** *Impact of speed on braking distance and risk of death. Sources: a) based on International Transport Forum (2012, p. 65) and b) Vivre en ville (2020, p. 3)*

Finally, let us mention that the emphasis placed on awareness and education campaigns intended to change pedestrian habits via the promotion of rule-abiding behavior is not justified by the inconclusive evaluation of such interventions. For example, the evaluation of three programs involving teaching pedestrian safety to children, adults and seniors found little or no effect on crosswalk behaviors (and decreasing effects over time), and no evidence of injury reduction (Duperrex et al. 2002; Celis-Morales et al. 2017; Twisk et al. 2014). These results remind us that the role of education is to generate public support and respect for more effective interventions to the built environment, but not to constitute a solution in itself.

#### 4.3.2.2. *The legislative context*

The greater or lesser risk of accidents is also associated with the actions taken at all government levels (from local to global) to protect pedestrians: better legislation and law enforcement (speed limits, drinking and driving bans, etc.), or more severe vehicle design standards and investment in trauma care (the implementation of an emergency medical treatment system). These actions have the potential to reduce the risk for all road users, including pedestrians. Ensuring mobility, while favoring potentially safer modes than the private car, such as collective transport, also makes up part of the legislative steps to be taken (Duduta et al. 2012).

#### 4.3.2.3. *The road and the built environment*

Beyond walkability indices, streets and intersections are also studied according to their propensity to limit or increase collision risks involving pedestrians. Characteristics such as heavy traffic or the presence of major roadways are known to increase collision rates (Dumbaugh and Li 2011; Morency et al. 2011; Maillot et al. 2017). By contrast, signalized intersections (stop signs, traffic lights) are known to reduce this risk (Rifaat et al. 2011; Rothman et al. 2014), as is the presence of buffer zones between the sidewalk and the road surface (Clifton et al. 2007; Negron-Poblete and Lord 2014; Paquin 2015) since these two elements separate pedestrians and vehicles in space and/or time.

For some years now, a body of work from developed countries has focused on traffic-calming measures. The purpose of these measures is to reduce vehicle volume and speed, thus creating more user-friendly living environments that are safer for walking (Bellefleur and Gagnon 2012). These measures are present in works on walkability and pedestrian safety, where changes to the geometry of streets and intersections (speed bumps, bottlenecks and chicanes, curb extensions, bollard narrowing lanes, etc.) are emphasized (Ewing 2001; Bunn et al. 2003; Retting et al. 2003; Tester et al. 2004; Jones et al. 2005; Clifton et al. 2007; Chaudhury et al. 2011;

Negron-Poblete and Lord 2014; Paquin 2015; Rothman et al. 2015; Lee and Dean 2018). A meta-analysis of traffic-calming interventions published in 2001 showed a 15% reduction in all collisions involving pedestrians, including a 25% reduction in collisions on residential streets (Elvik 2001). The general idea to grasp here is that an environment designed to slow cars down at crossing points (intersections, pedestrian crossings) or in neighborhoods (traffic-calming measures) limits the risk of error for drivers and generates a traffic flow that pedestrians can better understand and negotiate.

## 4.4. What interventions are needed to reduce collisions involving pedestrians and the severity of their injuries?

The WHO has estimated that half of road deaths could be prevented by implementing proven means already available in some places around the world (World Health Organization 2018b). Tackling road injuries by means of a Haddon matrix is instructive in many ways (Cloutier and Howard 2019).

The Haddon matrix is a concept dating back to the 1960s, used for describing actions that reduce the burden of injury (Haddon 1968). Haddon divided prevention into three stages: pre-crash, crash and post-crash. He also took into account the three components of a collision: the host (i.e. the injured victim), the agent (i.e. the vehicle involved and its driver) and the environment in which they interacted (including the road's physical environment, as well as its regulatory, social, legal and healthcare aspects). The combination of these three time periods with the three components results in a nine-cell matrix. Table 4.1 shows an example of a Haddon matrix for preventing pedestrian injuries and senior fatalities.

Let us mention that a large part of the success achieved in recent decades in terms of road safety is the result of improvements made to vehicles to better manage kinetic energy at the time of the collision (e.g. seat belts, airbags and vehicle roll cages). Nevertheless, this type of intervention aimed at protecting vehicle users does not benefit pedestrians. For the latter, interventions should focus on the pre-crash phase in order to reduce their occurrence at the source. The fact that interventions can be developed in each cell of the Haddon matrix implies a multidisciplinary and coordinated approach for creating pedestrian-friendly walking environments. This type of approach is also similar to the systemic vision of road safety implemented for over 20 years in Europe (in Sweden and the Netherlands, among others), and more recently in North America, as will be shown in the following section.

### 4.4.1. *Vision Zero: a systemic approach to road safety that can help with pedestrian safety*

Vision Zero, which originated in Sweden in 1997, offers a new paradigm for addressing road safety. The philosophy underlying this approach relies on the idea that the transport system must and can be designed to take into account the fact that humans will always make mistakes on the road (Vision Zero Network 2021). The design of this road system removes road safety responsibility from individuals, which will in turn lead to the removal of deaths and serious injuries, the "zero" degree to be achieved (Swedish Transportation Administration 2015).

The application of the Vision Zero approach requires the understanding that the built environment and the urban form can only be gradually changed, and that these changes are not exclusively determined by road safety requirements. On the other hand, road design and regulations are suitable for shorter-term changes. This is why the selection and prioritization of interventions must be based on local data (injuries, modes of transport, etc.) and on a coordinated approach that involves several actors working in complementary spheres (appointed officials, designers, engineers, police, public health experts, etc.) (Johansson 2009).

Based on a detailed analysis of conclusive data collected by a multidisciplinary team (urban planners, engineers, epidemiologists), the city of San Francisco drew up a pedestrian safety plan, a good empirical example of this approach (Kronenberg et al. 2015). On the other hand, the City of Montreal adopted the Vision Zero road safety plan in 2019, a promising project based on "thematic working groups" (TWGs) targeting behaviors and dangerous situations (speed, heavy vehicles, street-crossing), rather than user subgroups (Ville de Montréal 2020). The identification of 10 road safety "flaws" by these TWGs frames the 60 commitments in this plan, which should ultimately make it possible to improve the safety of pedestrians and all other road users.

| | Host (senior pedestrian) | Agent (vehicle and driver) | Environmental factors |
|---|---|---|---|
| **Pre-crash** | Walking training program to reduce the impact of (cognitive, mobility) deficits | Speed management (law implementation, police intervention to enforce the law)<br>Learning to drive | Traffic-calming measures<br>Speed limits<br>Road safety policy at national and local levels |
| **Crash** | Accompanying seniors on walks | Car design encouraging pedestrian protection (car hood) | Speed reduction ensured by urban planning |
| **Post-crash** | Access to low-cost healthcare and rehabilitation (public or private plan) | Evaluation of the effectiveness of the design on injuries<br>Violation tracking (black box for speed) | Access to a medical emergency service (ambulance or other)<br>Trauma hospital system |

**Table 4.1.** *Haddon matrix for senior pedestrians (source: Cloutier and Howard (2019), based on Haddon (1968))*

Although some criticize the utopian vision conveyed by the term "zero", we must admit that this approach is increasingly proving its worth, especially for pedestrians in big cities. For example, New York City has reported a 36% reduction in pedestrian fatalities since 2013 after adopting its Vision Zero plan (New York City Mayor's Office of Operations 2020). A Swedish study examining the evolution of pedestrian injuries between 2003 and 2017 showed a reduction in the likelihood of major road injuries after adopting the Vision Zero strategy and revealed that the increase in the number of walking seniors and active mobility policies are challenging for the authorities responsible for the road network, if this progress is to be sustained over time (Värnild et al. 2020). The same challenge is still faced by all dense urban environments.

### 4.4.2. *Reducing vehicle speed: an essential intervention for improving pedestrian mobility and safety*

As previously shown, the actual driving speed is related to the sign posted speed limit, a road risk in itself, especially for pedestrians. Interventions aimed at reducing speeds are therefore an essential way to improve the pedestrian experience and reduce the risk of injury and death. Speed reduction on roads can be achieved through a variety of interventions, including modifications to the built environment (traffic-calming measures, as already mentioned), regulatory changes (such as reduced speed limits) and effective law enforcement (e.g. automated speed control).

Despite being only few in number, the studies that have investigated the effects of speed limit reductions on pedestrian safety are unanimous, reporting a reduction in the number of pedestrians killed or seriously injured after the implementation of such reductions. For example, a Swiss study reflected a 16% reduction in car–pedestrian collisions, a 20% reduction in injuries and a 25% reduction in pedestrian fatalities after reducing the speed limit from 60 km/h to 50 km/h on urban streets (Waiz et al. 1983). Along the same lines, the study by Grundy et al. (2009) in the UK found that 20 mph (~32 km/h) speed zones were associated with a one-third reduction in pedestrian injuries, with greater reductions in children aged 0–15 years. More recently, a study conducted in the city of Toronto (Canada) associated the effect of lowering speed limits from 40 km/h to 30 km/h in neighborhoods with a 28% reduction in the incidence rate of collisions involving pedestrians, and a 67% reduction in major or fatal injuries of pedestrians involved in a collision after the speed limit change (Fridman et al. 2020).

Finally, automated speed control devices, including speed display boards and photo radars, are other interesting measures to reduce speeds on specific roads. A systematic review of 35 studies of photo radar showed reductions in average vehicle speed between 1% and 15%, and reductions in excessive speed between 14% and 65% (Wilson et al. 2010). In addition, the reductions before/after the installation of photo radars ranged from 8% to 49% for all collisions, and from 11% to 44% for fatal and serious injury collisions, all road users considered. Although the magnitude of the effect of such devices varies from study to study, they have all proven that photo radar is a valid tool for reducing road injuries.

However, reducing speed limits alone is not a guarantee of effectiveness compared to modifying roadway elements to encourage motorists to be more careful and to slow the speed at which they travel. Indeed, in a before/after study, Bellalite (2011) revealed that road users tend to significantly respect the sign posted speed limit when a change in the speed limit is accompanied by a change in the street layout and its surroundings (such as lane number, lane width, the presence of parking spaces on the street, a dense or high vegetation screen, etc.)

## 4.5. Avenues of research to improve pedestrian mobility

### 4.5.1. *Access to collision and exposure data to better portray pedestrian risk*

According to the Federal Highway Administration in the United States, data on collisions, traffic volume and road characteristics are required to be able to implement effective road safety interventions (Bellalite 2011; Sundstrom 2017). However, access to these three data sources presents a real challenge when it comes to collisions involving pedestrians (World Health Organization 2013). In fact, road risk for pedestrians (in terms of incidents, injuries and fatalities) is probably underestimated due to the lack of accurate data. For example, estimating the numerator (the total number of injured pedestrians) for the calculation of collision, injury or fatality rates can be difficult due to limitations in data sources (misclassifications or inaccuracies in location and time of collision; Imprialou and Quddus (2019)). Police reports and hospital records are the two main data sources for injured pedestrians. However, the under-reporting of this type of collision is well documented for police reports, especially for collisions involving less serious injuries (Janstrup et al. 2016; Doggett et al. 2018). In addition, in several jurisdictions, police reports and hospital records do not mention the location of the collision, which is crucial for developing effective interventions locally (Austin et al. 1997; Ahmadi et al. 2017).

Another significant data challenge relates to identifying accurate denominators for calculating risk rates. Data on pedestrian volumes rarely exist at the scale of streets and intersections. Surveys and household travel surveys (an alternative data source for pedestrian volumes) are only available at a larger territorial scale and with sometimes inadequate or incomplete walking information. When these data are used in combination with other modes of transport, it becomes cumbersome to extract data, even at this scale. Furthermore, these data sources make it possible to know the origin and the destination of the journeys, but not necessarily the route followed. Vehicle volume and speed data are collected more frequently, but are mostly available at traffic light intersections or on major roads where certain subgroups of pedestrians such as children tend not to walk (Rothman et al. 2019).

New methods for measuring exposure data (volume of vehicles and pedestrians) can accurately estimate the risk for pedestrians. Big data via the geolocation of mobile phones or even artificial intelligence/machine learning algorithms are likely to be promising (Yin et al. 2015; Nordback et al. 2016). However, exposure in terms of pedestrian volume or distance traveled (the risk per journey, whether reconstructed or known via GPS tracklogs) tends not to be considered when assessing the risk for pedestrians. This can lead to inconsistencies in diagnosing the extent of the problem and in the solutions offered to address it.

### 4.5.2. *The importance of assessing interventions and learning for the future*

Road safety strategies have historically been formulated around three "Es": engineering, education (or user awareness) and enforcement (police and legislative control). Lately, several other "Es" have appeared in road safety strategies, including "evaluation", which has been a relatively neglected element in recent decades. However, the evaluation of interventions using rigorous scientific methods is necessary to support evidence-based decision-making, one of the conditions for applying the Vision Zero strategy.

A meticulous evaluation of walking promotion interventions and of environmental changes is necessary for examining their effects on active transportation and/or pedestrian injuries. These evaluations should ideally involve randomized controlled trials, pre–post quasi-experimental and controlled studies (Stoker et al. 2015) and take into account the different scales of intervention (individuals, community) (Glasgow et al. 1999), which is not currently the case, with a few exceptions. These studies should take into account the differences between various subgroups of pedestrians, such as seniors or children (Dumbaugh and Frank 2007). For further details on intervention evaluation methods in relation to walking, see Chapter 5.

## 4.6. Conclusion

We are all pedestrians throughout our life stages and at different times of the day, whether schoolchildren going to school, adults or seniors for whom walking makes up part of their daily lives, or public transport users who walk to stations and stops. However, the availability of safe and comfortable pedestrian infrastructure is not evenly distributed throughout the different neighborhoods in cities, especially where the socio-economic status of populations varies, although the relationship between the two has not always been linear (Cowie et al. 2016; Bereitschaft 2017; Su et al. 2019). A report by the Organization for Economic Cooperation and Development (OECD) also points out that walking is still a forgotten mode of transport, barely taken into account during the planning process for transport and mobility (International Transport Forum 2012).

We should acknowledge the fact that the post-World War II urban model does not facilitate the task of actors who want to reinvent the city by and for pedestrians. In fact, the current configuration of the vast majority of the urban road network, except for a few areas downtown, is governed by an obligation to ensure the fluidity of automobile travel, to the point of inducing often excessive speeds for the most vulnerable users. Mobility plans highlighting "soft" modes of transport such as walking require political leadership, financial commitment and community recognition to deconstruct these configurations and imagine new ones. Conversely, the rallying call for the "war against cars" underlying some mobility plans, is, in our opinion, counterproductive. This rhetoric creates animosity among road users and stands in the way of the ultimate goal, which is keeping everyone safe, under all circumstances. After thoroughly reviewing research works on walkability, road risk and certain interventions required to mitigate it, this chapter has highlighted the main elements that need to be improved in our living environments, so that everyone can walk safely along the existing road network.

## 4.7. References

Adams, M.A., Frank, L.D., Schipperijn, J., Smith G., Chapman J., Christiansen L.B., Coffee N., Salvo, D., du Toit L., Dygrýn J. et al. (2014). International variation in neighborhood walkability, transit, and recreation environments using geographic information systems: The IPEN Adult Study. *International Journal of Health Geographics*, 13(43) 1–17.

Ahmadi, M., Valinejadi, A., Goodarzi, A., Safari, A., Hemmat, M., Majdabadi, H.A., Mohammadi, A. (2017). Geographic information system (GIS) capabilities in traffic accident information management: A qualitative approach. *Electronic Physician*, 9(6), 4533 4540.

Al Shammas, T. and Escobar, F. (2019). Comfort and time-based walkability index design: A GIS-based proposal. *International Journal of Environmental Research and Public Health*, 16(16), 2850.

Arason, N. (2014). *No Accident: Eliminating Injury and Death on Canadian Roads*. Wilfrid Laurier University Press, Waterloo.

Austin, K., Tight, M., Kirby, H. (1997). The use of geographical information systems to enhance road safety analysis. *Transportation Planning and Technology*, 20(3), 249–266.

Bélanger-Bonneau, H., Rannou, A., Thouez, J.-P., Damestoy, N. (2002). Les chutes à l'extérieur du domicile chez les personnes âgées de 55 ans et plus à Montréal et Laval. Report, Régie régionale de la santé et des services sociaux de Montréal-Centre, Direction de la santé publique, Montreal.

Bellalite, L. (2011). Étude des conditions optimales correspondant aux différentes limites de vitesse en milieu urbain. Report, Université de Sherbrooke, Laboratoire d'application et de recherche en aménagement, Quebec.

Bellefleur, O. and Gagnon, F. (2012). Apaisement de la circulation urbaine et santé : revue de littérature. Report, Centre de collaboration nationale sur les politiques publiques et la santé, INSPQ, Montreal.

Bereitschaft, B. (2017). Equity in neighbourhood walkability? A comparative analysis of three large U.S. cities. *Local Environment*, 22(7), 859–879.

Björnstig, U., Björnstig, J., Dahlgren, A. (1997). Slipping on ice and snow – Elderly women and young men are typical victims. *Accident Analysis & Prevention*, 29(2), 211–215.

Bunn, F., Collier, T., Frost, C., Ker, K., Roberts, I., Wentz, R. (2003). Traffic calming for the prevention of road traffic injuries: Systematic review and meta-analysis. *Injury Prevention*, 9(3), 200–204.

Celis-Morales, C.A., Lyall, D.M., Welsh, P., Anderson, J., Steell, L., Guo, Y., Maldonado, R., Mackay, D.F., Pell, J.P., Sattar, N. et al. (2017). Association between active commuting and incident cardiovascular disease, cancer, and mortality: Prospective cohort study. *BMJ*, 357(j1456). doi: 10.1136/bmj.j1456.

Cerin, E., Saelens, B.E., Sallis, J.F., Frank, L.D. (2006). Neighborhood environment walkability scale: Validity and development of a short form. *Medicine and Science in Sports and Exercise*, 38(9), 1682–1691.

Cervero, R. and Kockelman, K. (1997). Travel demand and the 3Ds: Density, diversity, and design. *Transportation Research Part D: Transport and Environment*, 2(3), 199–219.

Chaudhury, H., Sarte, A.F.I., Michael, Y.L., Mahmood, A., Keast, E.M., Dogaru, C., Wister, A. (2011). Use of a systematic observational measure to assess and compare walkability for older adults in Vancouver, British Columbia and Portland, Oregon neighbourhoods. *Journal of Urban Design*, 16(4), 433–454.

Clarke, P., Yan, T., Keusch, F., Gallagher, N.A. (2015). The impact of weather on mobility and participation in older US adults. *American Journal of Public Health*, 105(7), 1489–1494.

Clarke, P., Hirsch, J.A., Melendez, R., Winters, M., Sims Gould, J., Ashe, M., Furst, S., Mckay, H. (2017). Snow and rain modify neighbourhood walkability for older adults. *Canadian Journal on Aging*, 36(2), 159–169.

Clifton, K.J. and Livi, A.D. (2005). Gender differences in walking behavior, attitudes about walking, and perceptions of the environment in three Maryland communities. *Conference on Women's Issues in Transportation.* National Research Council (U.S.)/Transportation Research Board, Washington, 79–88.

Clifton, K.J., Livi Smith, A.D., Rodriguez, D. (2007). The development and testing of an audit for the pedestrian environment. *Landscape and Urban Planning*, 80 (1/2), 95–110.

Cloutier, M.-S. and Howard, A. (2019). Pedestrian injuries in cities. In *Handbook of Global Urban Health*, Vojnovic, I., Pearson, A.L., Asiki, G., DeVerteuil, G., Allen, A. (eds). Routledge, London.

Cloutier, M.-S., Beaulieu, E., Fridman, L., Macpherson, A.K., Hagel, B.E., Howard, A.W., Churchill, T., Fuselli, P., Macarthur, C., Rothman, L. (2021). State-of-the-art review: Preventing child and youth pedestrian motor vehicle collisions: Critical issues and future directions. *Injury Prevention*, 27(1), 77–84.

Cowie, C.T., Ding, D., Rolfe, M.I., Mayne, D.J., Jalaludin, B., Bauman, A., Morgan, G.G. (2016). Neighbourhood walkability, road density and socio-economic status in Sydney. *Environmental Health*, 15(1), 58.

Doggett, S., Ragland, D.R., Felschundneff, G. (2018). Evaluating research on data linkage to assess underreporting of pedestrian and bicyclist injury in police crash data. Research Report, UC Berkeley, Safe Transportation Research & Education Center [Online]. Available at: https://escholarship.org/content/qt0jq5h6f5/qt0jq5h6f5.pdf [Accessed 21 August 2020].

Dovey, K. and Pafka, E. (2020). What is walkability? The urban DMA. *Urban Studies*, 57(1), 93–108.

Duduta, N., Adriazola, C., Hidalgo, D., Lindau, L.A., Jaffe, R. (2012). Understanding road safety impact of high-performance bus rapid transit and busway design features. *Transportation Research Record*, 2317(1), 8–14.

Dumbaugh, E. and Frank, L. (2007). Traffic safety and safe routes to schools: Synthesizing the empirical evidence. *Transportation Research Record*, 2009(1), 89–97.

Dumbaugh, E. and Li, W. (2011). Designing for the safety of pedestrians, cyclists, and motorists in urban environments. *Journal of the American Planning Association*, 77(1), 69–88.

Duperrex, O., Bunn, F., Roberts, I. (2002). Safety education of pedestrians for injury prevention: A systematic review of randomized controlled trials. *BMJ*, 324, 1129–1133.

Elvik, R. (2001). Cost–benefit analysis of road safety measures: Applicability and controversies. *Accident Analysis & Prevention*, 33(1), 9–17.

Ewing, R. (2001). Impacts of traffic calming. *Transportation Quarterly*, 55(1), 33–46.

Ewing, R. and Cervero, R. (2010). Travel and the built environment. *Journal of the American Planning Association*, 76(3), 265–294.

Fenster, T. (2005). Gender and the city: The different formations of belonging. In *A Companion to Feminist Geography*, Nelson, L. and Seager, J. (eds). Blackwell Publishing, Malden.

Frank, L.D., Schmid, T.L., Sallis, J.F., Chapman, J., Saelens, B.E. (2005). Linking objectively measured physical activity with objectively measured urban form: Findings from SMARTRAQ. *American Journal of Preventive Medicine*, 28(2), 117–125.

Frank, L.D., Sallis, J.F., Saelens, B.E., Leary, L., Cain, L., Conway, T.L., Hess, P.M. (2010). The development of a walkability index: Application to the neighborhood quality of life study. *British Journal of Sports Medicine*, 44(13), 924–933.

Fridman, L., Ling, R., Rothman, L., Cloutier, M.S., Macarthur, C., Hagel, B., Howard, A. (2020). Effect of reducing the posted speed limit to 30 km per hour on pedestrian motor vehicle collisions in Toronto. Canada – A quasi experimental, pre-post study. *BMC Public Health*, 20(1), 56.

Gagné, M., Blanchet, C., Jean, S., Hamel, D. (2018). Chutes et facteurs associés chez les aînés québécois vivant à domicile. Report, Institut national de santé publique du Québec (INSPQ), Quebec.

Ghaffar, A., Hyder, A.A., Masud, T.I. (2004). The burden of road traffic injuries in developing countries: The 1st national injury survey of Pakistan. *Public Health*, 118(3), 211–217.

Giles-Corti, B., Macaulay, G., Middleton, N., Boruff, B., Bull, F., Butterworth, I., Badland, H., Mavoa, S., Roberts, R., Christian, H. (2014). Developing a research and practice tool to measure walkability: A demonstration project. *Health Promotion Journal of Australia*, 25(3), 160–166.

Glasgow, R.E., Vogt, T.M., Boles, S.M. (1999). Evaluating the public health impact of health promotion interventions: The RE-AIM framework. *American Journal of Public Health*, 89(9), 1322–1327.

Grundy, C., Steinbach, R., Edwards, P., Green, J., Armstrong, B., Wilkinson, P. (2009). Effect of 20 mph traffic speed zones on road injuries in London, 1986-2006: Control-led interrupted time series analysis. *BMJ*, 339 (b4469).

Guo, J.Y. and Gandavarapu, S. (2010). An economic evaluation of health-promotive built environment changes. *Preventive Medicine*, 50(1), S44–49.

Gyllencreutz, L., Björnstig, J., Rolfsman, E., Saveman, B.I. (2015). Outdoor pedestrian fall-related injuries among Swedish senior citizens injuries and preventive strategies. *Scandinavian Journal of Caring Sciences*, 29(2), 225–233.

Haddon, W. (1968). The changing approach to the epidemiology, prevention, and amelioration of trauma: The transition to approaches etiologically rather than descriptively based. *American Journal of Public Health and the Nation's Health*, 58(8), 1431–1438.

Haight, F.A. (1986). Risk, especially risk of traffic accident. *Accident Analysis & Prevention*, 18(5), 359–366.

Hakkert, A.S. and Braimaister, L. (2002). The uses of exposure and risk in road safety studies. Report, Institute for Road Safety Research (SWOV), Leidschendam.

Hauer, E. (1982). Traffic conflicts and exposure. *Accident Analysis & Prevention*, 14(5), 359–364.

Huguenin-Richard, F. and Cloutier, M.-S. (2021). Mesure du potentiel de marche et de l'accessibilité dans les espaces urbains pour les piétons âgés. *Flux*, 123(1), 30–53.

Huguenin-Richard, F., Granié, M.-A., Dommes, A., Coquelet, C., Cloutier, M.-S. (2014). La marche à pied pour les séniors : un mode de déplacement durable ? Report, Ministère de l'Écologie, de l'Énergie, du Développement durable et de la Mer, Paris.

Imprialou, M. and Quddus, M. (2019). Crash data quality for road safety research: Current state and future directions. *Accident Analysis & Prevention*, 130, 84–90.

International Transport Forum (2012). Piétons : sécurité, espace urbain et santé. Report, OECD Publishing, Paris.

International Transport Forum (2020). Road safety annual report 2020. Report, Paris.

Janstrup, K.H., Kaplan, S., Hels, T., Lauritsen, J., Prato, C.G. (2016). Understanding traffic crash underreporting: Linking police and medical records to individual and crash characteristics. *Traffic Injury Prevention*, 17(6), 580–584.

Johansson, R. (2009). Vision Zero – Implementing a policy for traffic safety. *Safety Science*, 47(6), 826–831.

Jones, S.J., Lyons, R.A., John, A., Palmer, S.R. (2005). Traffic calming policy can reduce inequalities in child pedestrian injuries: Database study. *Injury Prevention*, 11(3), 152–156.

Khanal, A. and Mateo-Babiano, I. (eds) (2016). What kind of built environment favours walking? A systematic review of the walkability indices. *Proceedings of the 38th Australasian Transport Research Forum*, Melbourne.

Kobusingye, O.C., Guwatudde, D., Lett, R. (2001). Injury patterns in rural and urban Uganda. *Injury Prevention*, 7, 46–50.

Kronenberg, C., Woodward, L., Dubose, B., Weissman, D. (2015). Achieving Vision Zero: Data-driven investment strategy to eliminate pedestrian fatalities on a city-wide level. *Transportation Research Record*, 2519(1), 146–156.

Labinjo, M., Juillard, C., Kobusingye, O.C., Hyder, A.A. (2009). The burden of road traffic injuries in Nigeria: Results of a population-based survey. *Injury Prevention*, 15(3), 157–162.

Lee, I.M. and Buchner, D.M. (2008). The importance of walking to public health. *Medicine and Science in Sports and Exercise*, 40(7), S512–518.

Lee, E. and Dean, J. (2018). Perceptions of walkability and determinants of walking behaviour among urban seniors in Toronto. *Journal of Transport and Health*, 9, 309–320.

Lee, S. and Talen, E. (2014). Measuring walkability: A note on auditing methods. *Journal of Urban Design*, 19(3), 368–388.

Lord, S. and Negron-Poblete, P. (2014). Les grands ensembles résidentiels adaptés québécois destinés aux aînés. Une exploration de la marchabilité du quartier à l'aide d'un audit urbain. *Norois*, 232, 35–52.

Maghelal, P.K. and Capp, C.J. (2011). Walkability: A review of existing pedestrian indices. *URISA Journal*, 23(2), 5–19.

Maillot, P., Dommes, A., Dang, N.T., Vienne, F. (2017). Training the elderly in pedestrian safety: Transfer effect between two virtual reality simulation devices. *Accident Analysis & Prevention*, 99A, 161–170.

Mammen, G. and Faulkner, G. (2013). Physical activity and the prevention of depression: A systematic review of prospective studies. *American Journal of Preventive Medicine*, 45(5), 649–657.

Morency, P., Gauvin, L., Tessier, F., Miranda-Moreno, L., Cloutier, M.S., Morency, C. (2011). Analyse désagrégée des facteurs environnementaux associés au nombre d'enfants blessés par un véhicule à moteur en milieu urbain. *Cahiers de Géographie du Québec*, 55(156), 449–468.

Moshiro, C., Heuch, I., Astrom, A.N., Setel, P., Hemed, Y., Kvale, G. (2005). Injury morbidity in an urban and a rural area in Tanzania: An epidemiological survey. *BMC Public Health*, 5(11).

Moura, F., Cambra, P., Gonçalves, A.B. (2017). Measuring walkability for distinct pedestrian groups with a participatory assessment method: A case study in Lisbon. *Landscape and Urban Planning*, 157, 282–296.

Mukhtar, M., Guillette, D., Lapos, N., Fitzpatrick, S., Jaros, R. (2019). An objective walkability index for public health and planning in Peel Region, Ontario, Canada. *Prev Chronic Dis.*, 16, E86 [Online]. Available at: https://www.cdc.gov/pcd/issues/2019/18_0469.htm [Accessed 4 April 2021].

Negron-Poblete, P. and Lord, S. (2014). Marchabilité des environnements urbains autour des résidences pour personnes âgées de la région de Montréal : application de l'audit MAPPA. *Cahiers de Géographie du Québec*, 58(164), 233–257.

New York City Mayor's Office of Operations (2020). Vision Zero: Year six report [Online]. Available at: https://www1.nyc.gov/assets/visionzero/downloads/pdf/vision-zero-year-6-report.pdf [Accessed 1 April 2021].

Nordback, K., Kothuri, S., Petritsch, T., Mcleod, P., Rose, E., Twaddell, H. (2016). Exploring pedestrian counting procedures: A review and compilation of existing procedures, good practices, and recommendations. Report, Federal Highway Administration, Washington.

Oxley, J., O'hern, S., Burtt, D., Rossiter, B. (2018). Falling while walking: A hidden contributor to pedestrian injury. *Accident Analysis & Prevention*, 114, 77–82.

Pabayo, R.A., Gauvin, L., Barnett, T.A., Morency, P., Nikiema, B., Seguin, L. (2012). Understanding the determinants of active transportation to school among children: Evidence of environmental injustice from the Quebec Longitudinal Study of Child Development. *Health & Place*, 18(2), 163–171.

Paquin, S. (2002). Pour un environnement urbain sécuritaire : guide d'aménagement. Report, Ville de Montréal, Montreal.

Paquin, S. (2015). Audit de potentiel piétonnier actif sécuritaire (PPAS) : le guide complet 2.1. Report, Direction de la santé publique, Montreal.

Public Health Agency of Canada. (2014). Seniors' Falls in Canada: Second Report. Report, Ottawa.

Quebec Board of the French Language (2009) Définition : marchabilité. Le grand dictionnaire terminologique [Online]. Available at: http://gdt.oqlf.gouv.qc.ca/ficheOqlf.aspx?Id_Fiche=8363771[Accessed 3 April 2021].

Raulin, F.O., Lord, S.B., Negron-Poblete, P. (2016). Évaluation de la marchabilité de trois environnements urbains de la région métropolitaine montréalaise à partir de l'outil MAPPA. *VertigO – la revue électronique en sciences de l'environnement*, 16(2), 1–30.

Retting, R.A., Ferguson, S.A., Mccartt, A.T. (2003). A review of evidence-based traffic engineering measures designed to reduce pedestrian–motor vehicle crashes. *American Journal of Public Health*, 93(9), 1456.

Rifaat, S., Tay, R., De Barros, A. (2011). Effect of street pattern on the severity of crashes involving vulnerable road users. *Accident Analysis & Prevention*, 43(1), 276–283.

Rothman, L., Buliung, R., Macarthur, C., To, T., Howard, A. (2014). Walking and child pedestrian injury: A systematic review of built environment correlates of safe walking. *Injury Prevention*, 20(1), 41–49.

Rothman, L., Macpherson, A., Buliung, R., Macarthur, C., To, T., Larsen, K., Howard, A. (2015). Installation of speed humps and pedestrian–motor vehicle collisions in Toronto, Canada: A quasi-experimental study. *BMC Public Health*, 15(74), 1–7.

Rothman, L., Cloutier, M.-S., Manaugh, K., Howard, A.W., Macpherson, A.K., Macarthur, C. (2019). Spatial distribution of roadway environment features related to child pedestrian safety by census tract income in Toronto, Canada. *Injury Prevention*, 26(3), 229–233.

Saelens, B.E., Sallis, J.F., Frank, L.D. (2003). Environmental correlates of walking and cycling: Findings from the transportation, urban design, and planning literatures. *Annals of Behavioral Medicine*, 25(2), 80–91.

Saghapour, T., Moridpour, S., Thompson, R.G. (2019). Estimating walking access levels incorporating distance thresholds of built environment features. *International Journal of Sustainable Transportation*, 13(1), 1–14.

Schepers, P., Den Brinker, B., Methorst, R., Helbich, M. (2017). Pedestrian falls: A review of the literature and future research directions. *Journal of Safety Research*, 62, 227–234.

Stockton, J.C., Duke-Williams, O., Stamatakis, E., Mindell, J.S., Brunner, E.J., Shelton, N.J. (2016). Development of a novel walkability index for London, United Kingdom: Cross-sectional application to the Whitehall II Study. *BMC Public Health*, 16(1), 1–12.

Stoker, P., Garfinkel-Castro, A., Khayesi, M., Odero, W., Mwangi, M.N., Peden, M., Ewing, R. (2015). Pedestrian safety and the built environment: A review of the risk factors. *Journal of Planning Literature*, 30(4), 377–392.

Su, S., Zhou, H., Xu, M., Ru, H., Wang, W., Weng, M. (2019). Auditing street walkability and associated social inequalities for planning implications. *Journal of Transport Geography*, 74, 62–76.

Sundstrom, C. (2017). Road safety fundamentals unit 3: Measuring safety. Report, Federal Highway Administration, Washington.

Swedish Transportation Administration (2015). Road safety – Vision Zero on the move [Online]. Available at: https://ec.europa.eu/transport/road_safety/sites/roadsafety/files/pdf/20151210_1_sweden.pdf [Accessed 4 April 2021].

Tester, J.M., Rutherford, G.W., Wald, Z., Rutherford, M.W. (2004). A matched case-control study evaluating the effectiveness of speed humps in reducing child pedestrian injuries. *American Journal of Public Health*, 94(4), 646–650.

Tournier, I., Dommes, A., Cavallo, V. (2016). Review of safety and mobility issues among older pedestrians. *Accident Analysis & Prevention*, 91, 24–35.

Transportation for America (2011). Dangerous by design: Solving the epidemic of preventable pedestrian deaths. Report, Washington.

Transportation for America (2021). Dangerous by design 2021. Report, National Complete Streets Coalition and Smart Growth America, Washington.

Twisk, D.A.M., Vlakveld, W.P., Commandeur, J.J.F., Shope, J.T., Kok, G. (2014). Five road safety education programmes for young adolescent pedestrians and cyclists: A multi-programme evaluation in a field setting. *Accident Analysis & Prevention*, 66, 55–61.

Vale, D.S., Saraiva, M., Pereira, M. (2016). Active accessibility: A review of operational measures of walking and cycling accessibility. *Journal of Transport and Land Use*, 9(1), 209–235.

Valentine, G. (1989). The geography of women's fear. *Area*, 21(4), 385–390.

Vargo, J., Stone, B., Glanz, K. (2012). Google walkability: A new tool for local planning and public health research? *Journal of Physical Activity and Health*, 9(5), 689–697.

Värnild, A., Tillgren, P., Larm, P. (2020). What types of injuries did seriously injured pedestrians and cyclists receive in a Swedish urban region in the time period 2003–2017 when Vision Zero was implemented? *Public Health*, 181, 59–64.

Vaughn, S.T. (2011). Women's safety and security issues with bicycling and walking: Examination of potential planning, design, and technology solutions. *Proceedings of the 4th International Conference on Women's Issues in Transportation*. National Research Council, Transportation Research Board, Washington.

Ville de Montréal (2020). État de la sécurité routière 2019. Report, Ville de Montréal, Montreal.

Vision Zero Network (2021). What is Vision Zero? [Online]. Available at: https://visionzeronetwork.org/about/what-is-vision-zero/ [Accessed 4 April 2021].

Vivre en ville (2020). Conception et mise en oeuvre de rues apaisées : outils pour concilier accessibilité, convivialité et sécurité sur les rues partagées et les rues étroites. Report, Vivre en Ville, Quebec.

Waiz, F.H., Hoefliger, M., Fehlmann, W. (eds) (1983). Speed limit reduction from 60 to 50 km/h and pedestrian injuries. *Proceedings of the 27th Stapp Car Crash Conference and Child Injury and Restraint Conference with IRCOBI*. SAE Technical Paper, San Diego.

Wilson, C., Willis, C., Hendrikz, J.K., Le Brocque, R., Bellamy, N. (2010). Speed cameras for the prevention of road traffic injuries and deaths. *Cochrane Database of Systematic Reviews*, 10, CD004607.

World Health Organization (2013). Pedestrian safety: A road safety manual for decision-makers and practitioners. Report, WHO, Geneva.

World Health Organization (2018a). Les chutes. Report, WHO, Geneva [Online]. Available at: https://www.who.int/fr/news-room/fact-sheets/detail/falls [Accessed 1 April 2021].

World Health Organization (2018b). Rapport de situation sur la sécurité routière dans le monde 2018. Report, WHO, Geneva [Online]. Available at: https://www.who.int/violence_injury_prevention/road_safety_status/2018/French-Summary-GSRRS2018.pdf [Accessed 3 April 2021].

Yin, L., Cheng, Q., Wang, Z., Shao, Z. (2015). "Big data" for pedestrian volume: Exploring the use of Google street view images for pedestrian counts. *Applied Geography*, 63, 337–345.

# 5

# The Geographical Dimension of Daily Active Mobility

**Thierry FEUILLET[1,2] and Hélène CHARREIRE[3,4,5]**
[1] *IDEES, Université de Caen, France*
[2] *EREN, Université Sorbonne Paris Nord, Bobigny, France*
[3] *MoISA, Cirad, CIHEAM-IAMM, INRAE, Institut Agro, IRD, Université de Montpellier, France*
[4] *Lab'URBA, Université Paris-Est Créteil, France*
[5] *Institut universitaire de France, Paris, France*

## 5.1. Introduction

Active mobility (which mainly concerns the practice of walking and cycling) represents a particularly interesting lever for combating physical inactivity and its associated health problems, insofar as it is an important component of physical activity and can be practiced routinely and on a daily basis. The links between physical activity and health are well known: there are clear causal associations between increased physical activity and reduced morbidity and mortality from cardiovascular and respiratory diseases and mental health disorders (Sallis et al. 2012). Active mobility, which does not generate pollutant emissions, is also part of sustainable mobility dimensions, respecting the main goals of sustainable development (and thus contributing to social and economic well-being, without damaging the environment or human health). The transitional pandemic context after Covid-19, which profoundly altered our daily mobility habits and practices, can also serve as an opportunity to develop walking and cycling behaviors. Indeed, social distancing rules imposed by many governments limited the use of collective

*Everyday Mobility and Health*,
coordinated by Julie VALLÉE. 

modes of transport in favor of individual ones, in part represented by active mobility.

Encouraging active mobility in daily life requires studying its determinants, in particular those related to the environment, since they are potentially modifiable by urban planners at the local level. This is especially the case in urban areas, where shorter average travel distances are potentially better suited for active modes of transport. For example, according to CEREMA, in French urban areas nearly 10% of journeys made by car are shorter than 1 km – which approximately represents a 15-minute walk – while 4 trips out of 10 are shorter than 3 km (CEREMA 2015). These short-distance journeys in urban areas offer the potential for a modal shift from the car to active modes of transport. With a focus on the city, this chapter will discuss this carryover potential. While these questions may be similar to the ones arising in peripheral or rural areas, the challenges relating to daily travel over longer distances are not the same.

Although the links between places and health-related behaviors are now better known, their complexity continues to feed the reflection of researchers in geography and in public health more than ever (Dixon et al. 2021). For several years, geographers and epidemiologists have made it clear that many aspects of the built environment, such as cycling and pedestrian amenities, the presence and quality of sidewalks, shop density, neighborhood aesthetics, etc., influence active mobility to a certain extent. An inventory of these environmental characteristics in relation to walking and cycling will be presented in the first section of this chapter.

Nevertheless, these links between environmental characteristics and active mobility may vary depending on the territorial context. In other words, the effects of the environmental determinants of mobility are spatially differentiated. The territorial heterogeneity of environmental effects on behaviors is rarely studied, even though it reveals mechanisms closely related to the local specificities of territories (context effects) and the way in which places and people co-construct one another. A better understanding of these local specificities could constitute a valuable source of information for public decision-makers and urban planners in charge of designing the cities of the future. Hence, the second section of the chapter (section 5.3) will be devoted to the question of context effects and their role in producing territorial heterogeneity, as observed via active mobility.

Recently, in situ experiments have measured the impact of urban planning (e.g. continuity of pedestrian routes, cycling lanes, public transport stations, modification of traffic plans) on individual behaviors, by following a rigorous methodological protocol. These longitudinal experiments provide the keys to understanding causal relationships between the urban planning of new environments and behavioral changes, especially in active mobility. The third and last section of the chapter (section 5.4) will be dedicated to urban experimentation evaluation studies in different territorial contexts around the world. The chapter will conclude (section 5.5) with the challenges represented by development strategies on active mobility, and more broadly, on health and socio-spatial health inequalities.

## 5.2. Environment and active mobility: what is the relationship?

Despite the scientific evidence on the relationship between physical activity (including active mobility) and health status, the practice of physical activity in the general population (adults and adolescents) decreases while sedentariness increases, both in the professional context and during leisure time and daily travel (SPF 2017). Regardless of their occupational activity, the proportion of French adults who report spending 3 hours or more in front of a screen each day increased from 53% in 2006 to 80% in 2015. On the contrary, the modal share of walking (number of journeys) gradually decreased, from 33.7% in 1982 to 23.2% in 1994 and 22.3% in 2008, before experiencing a slight recent increase to 23.7% in 2019 (Ministry of Ecological Transition 2019).

It is necessary to question the characteristics and representations of the contexts in which activities are performed to better understand how these contexts facilitate or, on the contrary, limit the practice of physical activity, especially walking and cycling. The context in which an individual evolves – today considered a determinant of physical activity behaviors – is defined by the elements of the built environment (transport networks, land use, green spaces, etc.), which is itself associated with the socio-economic level of the neighborhood or municipality (median income or level of social disadvantage, for example).

Thus, the practice of walking or cycling for the daily commute depends on the characteristics and capacities specific to each individual and on varied factors such as urbanization, land use and urban infrastructure (Sallis and Glanz 2006).

### 5.2.1. *Characterizing the urban context*

In the international literature, the characteristics of the context (see Box 5.1 for a discussion of the geographical delimitation of these contexts) have been analyzed separately or combined into synthetic indicators, for example, in the form of walkability (pedestrian or walkability index) and cycling potential (bikeability).

The work of Frank et al. (2005), in the city of Atlanta (United States), initially defined walkability as the combination of three variables: residential density, the density of intersections on a street grid and the mix of land uses, these three variables being assumed as positively associated with walking.

An important research issue regarding the links between environment and active mobility lies in defining the exposure area, that is, all the areas destined for walking and cycling practices. In the majority of works, the neighborhood of residence is used as the unique exposure area in the urban context, defined by administrative boundaries or by an area centered around the place of residence.

However, very few people know the administrative boundaries of their neighborhood of residence, and even fewer who only travel within those boundaries or in a predefined space (apart from exceptional periods such as the lockdown in Spring 2020 due to the Covid-19 crisis), immediately limiting the scope of empirical results (Petrović et al. 2020). Kwan (2012) referred to the problems regarding the delimitation of the exposure context as "The Uncertain Geographic Context Problem".

Recently, new approaches have been proposed for defining the neighborhood boundaries as perceived by inhabitants (Vallée et al. 2015; Charreire et al. 2016) or for defining the activity space taking into account all of the areas of daily life (Perchoux et al. 2013, 2019). These innovative approaches promote an idiosyncratic vision of the exposure context, encompassing all individual characteristics.

**Box 5.1.** *Defining the geographical exposure area*

For over 15 years, the pedestrian and cycling potential have inspired multiple definitions (notably for the former) and various measures combining different objective and subjective criteria, such as the density of equipment and/or services, the diversity of uses, the density of road networks, of intersections or even the feeling of security, the aesthetics or the cleanliness of facilities. For example, several walkability indices have been developed to assess the walkability of North American[1] cities. We can mention the Pedestrian Environment Data Scan (PEDS, Clifton et al. 2007), defined on the basis of 31 criteria, the Irvine–Minnesota Inventory, which takes into account 162 criteria (Day et al. 2006), or the walkability index for seniors (MAPPA) proposed in Canada (Raulin et al. 2016).

More recently, this type of measure has been developed in certain European countries (Grasser et al. 2017). In France, the *Direction régionale et interdépartementale de l'équipement et de l'aménagement* (DRIEA) from Île-de-France developed a fine-scale walkability index (400 m grid) taking into account sidewalk length, the surface of vegetation and the distance to downtown Paris (DRIEA 2019).

### 5.2.2. *The multidimensional determinants of active mobility*

In general terms, the practice of walking and cycling is more important in areas characterized by high walkability, the proximity and density of public transport networks, shops, local services and green spaces, as well as quality walking and cycling infrastructures (Saelens and Handy 2008; Ewing and Cervero 2010; Giles-Corti et al. 2016). Ewing and Cervero (2010) grouped these characteristics under five "Ds" (density, design, destinations, diversity and distances), bearing in mind that, in this classification, elements are interdependent. The environment's representations in relation to aesthetics, the feeling of safety or transportation modes are also determinants of active mobility and, more particularly, of walking (in the context of commuting and of recreational trips).

The influence of the environment on active mobility may vary depending on the mode (walking, cycling) and the reason for traveling (work, leisure). For example, the density of amenities and green spaces in the neighborhood of residence are specifically associated with so-called recreational walking (during leisure time), whereas land use diversity tends to be associated with utilitarian walking (i.e. walking aimed towards a destination) (Saelens and Handy 2008; McCormack and Shiell 2011; Chaix et al. 2014). Let us consider the Canadian case: while the neighborhood's level of walkability influences the practice of walking to work, the impact on recreational walking seems to be less obvious. Another example, related to cycling, is drawn from the work

1. See: https://activelivingresearch.org.

of Yang et al. (2019). This team analyzed the results of 39 articles, published between 2007 and 2017 and addressing built environment–cycling relationships. The results showed that while the high connectivity of the road network and the presence of amenities and cycling lanes increase the practice of cycling to work, these relationships are not significant for recreational cycling.

In an international study (International Physical activity and Environment Network – IPEN), conducted among 14,000 adults (between 18 and 66 years old) within 17 cities and across 12 countries between 2002 and 2011, the population density, the intersections and the number/proximity of parks in the neighborhoods of residence were positively associated with the inhabitants' walking practice (min/week), regardless of the method used for assessing built environment indicators (either objectively through a geomatic approach or based on statements reflecting the people's perception) (Sallis et al. 2020). The neighborhoods in which the subjects reported the presence of pedestrian infrastructure and identified them as attractive from an aesthetic point of view matched those in which the practice of walking was widespread (regardless of the walkers' origin). However, other studies have stressed the inconsistency of this link from country to country, in particular when the environment's characterization (aesthetics, feeling of security, road network connectivity, residential density, cycling facilities) is based on what the participants have reported.

The results of 42 studies estimating the associations between the (objective and perceived) characteristics of the residential environment and active transportation modes (walking and cycling) among people over 65 were analyzed (Cerin et al. 2017). For this population category, in addition to the characteristics identified for the general population (density of services/shops, public transport, etc.), the presence of sidewalks with well-maintained surfaces (to avoid the risk of falling) and places to rest (benches) along the route was positively associated with the practice of walking. As regards cycling, the authors observed that relationships were by far heterogeneous and remained practically understudied in people over 65 (five studies combined walking and cycling and two Belgian studies only focused on cycling (Van Cauwenberg et al. 2012; Van Holle et al. 2014)).

As far as international studies are concerned, associations are less clear and frequent between the (measured or reported) characteristics of the built environment and certain health indicators, such as the body mass index (BMI) or the prevalence of overweight people (IPEN, International Physical activity and Environment Network). However, these previous analyses are mainly based on cross-sectional studies, which end up being unsuitable for understanding long-term pathologies and chronic disorders such as obesity or diabetes. On the contrary, Chandrabose et al. (2019) have recently conducted a meta-analysis of 36 longitudinal studies according to which walkability in the neighborhood of residence was the characteristic most frequently associated with the incidence of obesity, type-2 diabetes and hypertension (Chandrabose et al. 2019). Although some characteristics of the residential environment seem to be more frequently associated with active mobility, the relationships observed in the literature are highly variable – even contradictory – depending on the populations studied, the nature of control variables, the indicators used for quantifying the environment and for measuring walking and cycling (James et al. 2014; Strominger et al. 2016; Peters et al. 2020).

The results of these studies – briefly summarized in this section – are difficult to generalize to all countries, whose investments in terms of urban and transport policies, as well as the representations of active transport modes, can vary greatly. This also happens between different regions within the same country. This question of the relationships between urban context and active mobility has attracted particular attention in North American cities (strongly marked by urban sprawl, by the predominance of car use and the scarcity of pedestrian and cycling infrastructure), in Australian cities and in large metropolitan areas in Europe. In Europe, aspects such as access to recreational facilities, aesthetic considerations and criminality indicators do not seem to be associated with walking and cycling practices, whereas these characteristics are more present in North American studies (Van Holle et al. 2012).

Research still needs to be developed in order to analyze these relationships in medium-sized cities, in peripheral or even rural areas, as well as in middle- and low-income countries, for which studies are almost non-existent (Elshahat et al. 2020). Significant differences can appear even at the scale of one city. Therefore, we should not focus so much on the characteristics significantly and systematically associated with active mobility (irrespective of urban forms, population or country profiles), but identify levers and potential obstacles to the practice of walking and cycling at each local context.

In this sense, the analysis of the territorial heterogeneity of relationships between the environment and active mobility represents a relevant entry point for targeting and understanding local contexts and for optimizing the potential interventions that will be implemented.

## 5.3. Territorial heterogeneity of the relationship between living environment and active mobility: the importance of context effects

Depending on the location, environmental characteristics may not have the same effects on the individuals' active mobility behavior or, broadly speaking, their health. While the presence of many wide sidewalks downtown may encourage some individuals to walk more, is this applicable to sparsely populated neighborhoods without shops? Or to neighborhoods marked by demographic or socio-economic characteristics? The spatial co-occurrences of certain environmental amenities, associated with the characteristics of the populations who frequent such areas, produce singular associations that are geographically heterogeneous[2] in essence. The complexity of these mechanisms and their effects on behavior and health has long led to these areas being regarded as black boxes, animated by mysterious "social miasmas" (Macintyre et al. 2002). A clearer theoretical standpoint is needed to better appraise local variations in the environment–individual behavior links. In this way, a possible reading of these spatial variations in environment–behavior relationships would be to consider that they result from a set of mechanisms grouped under the concept of context effects. In simplified terms, these can be defined as the specific effects of a group of observations regarding a specific area (without an a priori defined scale). Drawing inspiration from the typologies of Manski (1993) and Galster (2012), two major mechanisms operating within spatial contexts can be mentioned (Feuillet 2021).

The first of these mechanisms concerns effects occurring exclusively within the context, and which can therefore be described as endogenous. On the one hand, these endogenous effects result from social interactions between individuals related by their geographical proximity, which can promote a convergence of behaviors, via contagion processes, for example. This will especially be observed in particular at the local scale, the street or the neighborhood. On the other hand, a convergence of behaviors can also occur due to shared exposure to local norms or specificities, without the need for social interactions. These local standards may arise from the particular co-occurrence of environmental characteristics (e.g. via the presence of

2. Associations between environmental amenities and mobility behavior can also be *temporally* heterogeneous. They can vary depending on the seasons, the days of the week or the time of day (Vallée 2017). However, this temporal heterogeneity of the relationships between living environment and active mobility will not be detailed here.

secure cycling facilities in combination with infrastructure that restricts car use), contributing to the specificity of a place and influencing behavior in a particular way. They can also result from the implementation of local public policies, aimed at promoting health in a way that caters to different territorial needs (districts, cities, regions or even countries).

The second mechanism includes exogenous effects, those involving the proximity of contexts, their location in a larger territorial system. Thus, the position of a neighborhood in the hierarchy of the urban system – downtown, the suburbs or the peri-urban belt – and the spatial interactions linking this neighborhood to its neighbors, contribute to a better understanding of the heterogeneous relationships between the different territories. For example, the distance to the main employment areas, to urban centers, the forces of attractiveness or repulsion of neighboring districts, can explain the variable effect of infrastructure on active mobility, even in "intrinsically" similar neighborhoods. Applying these hypotheses to obesity, Feuillet et al. (2020) showed that the relationship between the social disadvantage of the neighborhood of residence and the risk of being overweight is higher in the suburbs of large cities than downtown or in rural areas. This illustrates the effect of the position of context in its territorial system.

The existence of these spatial contexts partly explains the spatial heterogeneity of environment–active mobility relationships revealed by numerous empirical studies, regardless of the variability of methodological protocols (choice of quantification of environments and behaviors and choice of modeling methods).

For example, within the same metropolitan area (the Seoul agglomeration), Kim et al. (2019) showed that the effects of the built environment (sidewalk width, road density, distance to public transport) on the volume of pedestrians varied depending on the neighborhood, reflecting correlations that were sometimes positive, sometimes negative or even non-existent in some places. In the Paris region, working on a sample of nearly 5,000 adults from the Nutrinet-Santé cohort, Feuillet et al. (2016) revealed that the effect of the built environment (shop density, residential density) on walking (utilitarian as well as recreational) was stronger in the northern half of Paris than in the rest of the inner suburbs. Similarly, Cheng et al. (2021) mapped local nuances in the relationships between the walking time of the elderly and the built environment in Nanjing, China, including sign reversals (in particular for the effect of population density and urban land use diversity).

At the regional scale, working on a sample of 40,000 French adults, Feuillet et al. (2018) also showed that the spatial heterogeneity of built environment–active mobility relationships could be observed between cities and regions. For example, while the probability of walking for a utilitarian purpose markedly increases with a dense vegetation cover in the lower Rhône valley and in Normandy, it does so very little in the Paris region or in Brittany. Regarding the relationship between the (social or built) environment and obesity, similar results have been reported in the scientific literature at the local scale (Faka et al. 2019; Oshan et al. 2020) as well as at the regional scale (Wen et al. 2010; Chen and Truong 2012; Myers et al. 2015; Lee et al. 2019; Feuillet et al. 2020) and in different regions worldwide.

Moreover, the theoretical mechanisms governing the above-mentioned context effects are likely to overlap, to combine and must be considered under an environment–health relational approach, that is, without a unidirectional effect (Cummins et al. 2007) and without the possibility of differentiating them strictly through observation. Places influence behavior just as much as human beings build places, places that are always interacting within a larger territorial system that influences them in return.

Considered in a purely quantitative way, this spatial heterogeneity emerging from empirical studies necessarily reflects poor quantification or the failure to take into account local environmental characteristics. A first possible line of research could start by questioning the relevance and construction of environmental indicators likely to capture these local specificities, and whose inclusion in the models would remove spatial heterogeneity and facilitate the generalization of results. Another avenue of research could involve identifying the common features among spaces with similar effects in meaning and intensity. The interpretation of these effects' heterogeneity would be facilitated.

In any case, this spatial heterogeneity has important implications in terms of public health. It implies that the effectiveness of a particular policy for encouraging health-promoting behaviors (such as active mobility) is likely to vary locally in response to context effects. This observation should encourage us to give priority to local studies in research, rather than those solely oriented towards the observation of average relationships across the whole of a territory. This vision also corroborates the fact that in France, it is mainly at the local scale (municipalities and inter-communalities) that public stakeholders have the opportunity to act on the built environment to promote active mobility practices.

Beyond the question of spatial heterogeneity, analysis of the environment–active mobility relationship should also be favored in the context of longitudinal studies to better appreciate the impact of different contexts throughout the life of individuals and to try to establish causal links. These longitudinal analyses would make it possible to acknowledge urban modifications or transformations or even to assess their impact on active mobility.

## 5.4. From the promotion of active mobility in public health to health-enhancing urban planning

A lever for modifying health-related mobility behaviors – active modes – could involve acting on the living contexts of populations, and more particularly, modifying urban characteristics (Giles-Corti et al. 2016). While redeveloping the city to meet mobility, health and well-being issues is not new, the assessment of the impact of these developments on behavior, and more broadly on health, is still insufficient to clarify and guide urban planning decisions (Ogilvie et al. 2020). These evaluations are still scarce because they require specific methods, integrating long time periods, at different scales, and cross-views between researchers from different disciplines, operational stakeholders and populations.

For example, low emission zones (LEZ – which limit the entry of vehicles to all or part of the city and/or penalizes the most polluting vehicles) have been developed since the 2000s in many European cities, with the aim of improving air quality. However, Mudway et al. (2019) pointed out that despite the political and financial costs of these LEZ, retrospective evaluation studies on the effectiveness of these policies on health are scant. The impact of these LEZ and of other urban transformations can vary considerably depending on the socio-economic characteristics of the populations and the spatial contexts (see section 5.2) and can, in some cases, lead to a deterioration of health behaviors (active mobility) and an increase in social health inequalities. The expression "urban transformations" comprises a set of processes ranging from the definition of an urban planning project to its completion, and also involves phases of community consultation and more or less important modifications. These transformations can take the form of "simple" road development operations (sidewalk widening, for example) as well as large-scale operations within the framework of neighborhood renewal or renovation. In France, these dimensions fall under the responsibility of the *Agence nationale pour la rénovation urbaine* (ANRU, National Agency for Urban Renewal).

### 5.4.1. *Evaluating the impact of urban changes on active mobility practices and representations*

In many disciplines (medicine, epidemiology, etc.), in order to assess whether changes in behavior or health outcomes are directly attributable to an intervention (causality), two groups are compared: those having received the intervention and those who have not.

Randomized controlled trials (RCT) make it possible to meet this goal through:

– researcher control of the intervention;

– randomization (draw), which involves randomly distributing the groups (intervention and control/reference group).

This random distribution ensures the initial comparability (before the intervention) of groups by guaranteeing that all the prognostic or determining factors (whether known or not) are fairly distributed between the two groups. However, this type of study in which one chooses a priori to intervene on one group and not on another (known as the control group) can be difficult, even impossible to carry out due to economical, practical or ethical reasons.

Therefore, researchers have turned to so-called quasi-experimental studies (Petticrew 2011). This design refers to an experiment based on a controlled intervention (in an experimental room or in the context of trials) and two groups, but without resorting to randomization. When the intervention takes place under "real" (uncontrolled) conditions, we speak of a natural experiment (Leatherdale 2019). The Medical Research Council in the UK has defined "natural experimentation" as the events, interventions or policies that have not been manipulated by researchers but are still amenable to research and rely on the exposure variation they generate to evaluate impacts (Craig et al. 2012). This type of study requires a longitudinal before/after (the intervention) design with a reference site contemporary with the intervention, in order to limit the selection bias between populations.

**Box 5.2.** *Which methods to evaluate urban interventions?*

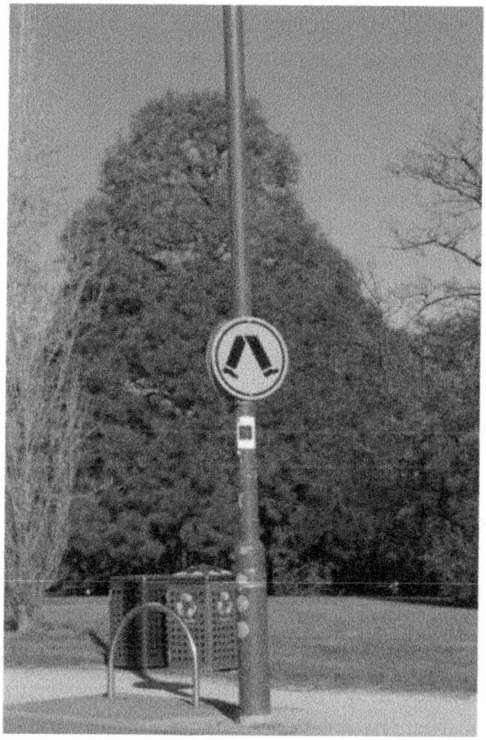

a)

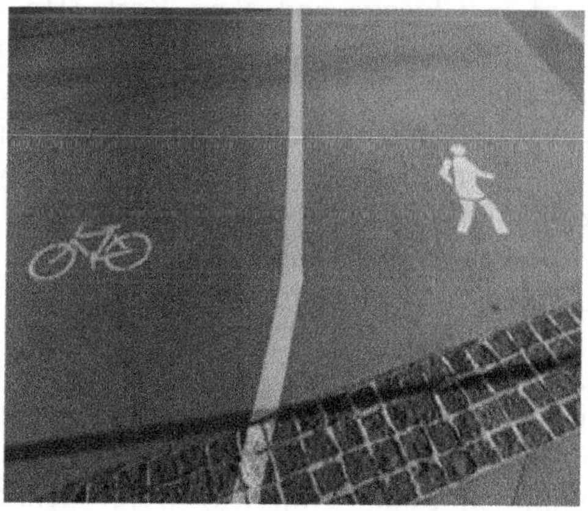

b)

**Figure 5.1.** *Examples of urban signage systems dedicated to active mobility on the streets of Melbourne, Australia (May 2011, H. Charreire). For a color version of this figure, see www.iste.co.uk/vallee/everyday.zip*

As regards the evaluation methodologies (see Box 5.2), different study designs can be implemented, depending on the target population and the research questions, each with their own advantages and disadvantages (see Craig et al. 2013; Leatherdale 2019; Tharrey 2020). Let us emphasize that development of such experiments for analyzing the impact of urban transformations (e.g. the creation or renewal of public transport infrastructure or green spaces) on physical activity practices, including walking and cycling, is rare. In our area of interest, natural experiment studies aim to assess the change in physical activity attributable to a specific intervention, such as the creation or redevelopment of cycling lanes, walking paths, green spaces or gardens, urban signage systems and infrastructures (Figures 5.1 and 5.2), or broader redevelopments, as part of urban renewal projects. Some examples of this type of study are shown in Figure 5.1.

In 2009, the island of Montreal was equipped with a public bicycle sharing system (BIXI©, a contraction of BIcylce-taXI), whose impact on cycling was assessed immediately after it was set up (May to June 2009), a few months later (October to December 2009) and 18 months later (October to December 2010) in two population groups divided according to the distance between their place of residence and a BIXI station (more or less 500 m) (Fuller et al. 2013). While the impact seemed limited the first year of the intervention, the results showed a significant increase in the practice of cycling during the second year for those living nearby stations. Similar results were observed in Chicago and New York (Hosford et al. 2019). Panter et al. (2019) identified and analyzed 13 "natural experiments" whose developments focused on the creation of new walking and cycling paths (seven studies), cycling lanes (five studies) and the setting up of cycling infrastructure, in this case Montreal's BIXI (one study). Five of them identified favorable changes in the direction of an increase in active mobility or of physical activity in general. The other studies did not reveal any change in the behaviors studied.

In another systematic review published in 2018 (MacMillan et al. 2018), 15 articles evaluating the impact of urban development on physical activity and/or diet (ten in the United States, three in the United Kingdom, one in New Zealand and one in South America) were identified. Five studies focused on the impact of the creation/redevelopment of cycling lanes and the continuity of pedestrian routes, two of which also included green spaces, four studied the establishment of new stops or public transport lines and four analyzed the effects of setting up new shops. Eight of them observed positive changes in physical activity and diet.

In France, public health research based on "natural experiments" is at an embryonic stage. A recent study carried out as part of the JArDinS (*Jardins urbains pour une Alimentation Durable et Saine*, Urban Gardens for Sustainable and Healthy Food) project has made it possible to measure the potential impact of participation in a shared garden in the city of Montpellier to encourage the adoption of a more favorable and healthy lifestyle, especially in terms of food (e.g. the nutritional quality of supplies, sensitivity to food waste) and physical activity (Tharrey et al. 2019). At the end of the first year, researchers did not observe any changes in the behavior of (new) gardeners who decided to join the shared garden in 2018 (Tharrey 2020). However, this first exploration has identified a certain discouragement on the part of these (neo)gardeners in the face of the difficulties encountered (lack of time and knowledge in gardening, conflicts, distance). On the contrary, the authors of previous experiments (e.g. BIXI on cycling) observed changes only after the second year of the intervention and insisted on the need to carry out measurements over long periods of time.

At a larger scale, Kramer et al. (2014) analyzed recreational activity practices (walking, cycling, sport) before and after the implementation of urban renewal operations in 40 disadvantaged neighborhoods in the Netherlands. Evaluation after three years showed a significant increase in recreational walking in the renovated neighborhoods in comparison with the others. Such changes, however, did not apply to recreational cycling or sports activities (Kramer et al. 2014, 2017). In London, three outer boroughs (Waltham Forest, Kingston, Enfield) have benefited since 2016 from the "Mini-Hollands" program, which aims to modify the urban environment to make it more favorable to active modes of transport through a wide variety of measures ranging from the redevelopment of public space (cycling lanes, street furniture) to the organization of events to promote these activities. Aldred et al. (2021) observed an approximate 40-minute increase per week in active mobility practices (walking, in particular) for the inhabitants of the districts having benefited from significant investments within the program's framework, compared to the inhabitants from other boroughs, and more generally, from London. In Canada, the INTERACT (*INTErventions urbaines, Recherche-Action, Communautés et sanTé*, Urban Interventions, Action-Research, Community and Health) team is currently evaluating the impact of urban changes on health and well-being in the neighborhoods of cities such as Montreal, Vancouver, Victoria and Saskatoon (Kestens et al. 2019). The first results observed in the city of Montreal and Vancouver showed that the residents surveyed – namely in central neighborhoods – reported that their urban environment had improved, facilitating active modes and having a positive effect on their quality of life.

From this first synthesis, two main questions remain. Firstly, while the transformations carried out within the framework of urban renewal operations seemed to have significant effects on health-related behaviors (physical activity, in particular), the impact of specific amenities remains variable, as a number of studies have shown. For instance, how and why does a new amenity such as the creation of a new cycling or pedestrian path seem to impact active mobility in certain neighborhoods or cities, but does not do so systematically? As previously mentioned (section 5.2), place effects (the effects of local spatial co-occurrences having certain environmental characteristics, or social interactions within specific urban contexts) play a major role in the heterogeneity of these impacts. Secondly, the potentially negative impact of these amenities, and of redevelopment and renovation operations in particular, has been scarcely explored from the point of view of health inequalities. Do these amenities favor active mobility for the entire population or, on the contrary, do they contribute to widening inequalities by mainly targeting the most well-off populations and/or by modifying the social composition of neighborhoods towards gentrification (Gibbons et al. 2018; Izenberg et al. 2018; Angelovski et al. 2020; Bhavsar et al. 2020)?

### 5.4.2. *Active mobility and physical activity in the time of Covid-19*

The epidemic context the world has been experiencing since the beginning of 2020 caused a profound change in individual mobility practices, a change that is still in progress at the time of writing. The first effect of coronavirus on individual mobility translated to an overall decrease in journeys and distances traveled (Abdullah et al. 2020), especially during strict lockdown periods. In France, for example, the number of trips decreased by 65% during the spring of 2020 (Pullano et al. 2020).

Public transport was the modal choice most impacted by this decrease, due to the short distance between individuals (Gkiotsalitis and Cats

2021). Several governments, as well as the WHO, explicitly advocated avoiding the choice of public transport as much as possible. Tirachini and Cats (2020) calculated changes in the use of public transport in 10 countries between March and June 2020 based on Google[3] mobility data, revealing that nine of those countries recorded a drop of over 40% in this mode, reaching 80% in Italy. In Chicago, the use of public transport decreased by 72% (Hu and Chen 2021). This abandonment of public transport raised the key question as to the nature of modal shifts. A high risk of a modal shift towards private cars was observed (Honey-Rosés et al. 2020), an unfavorable solution both in terms of public health (physical inactivity) and environmental externalities (greenhouse gas emissions). For example, this was the case in Australia (Beck et al. 2020), and the same was observed by Abdullah et al. (2020), who worked with a sample of 1,200 people in different countries.

However, the context of a sudden change also represented a remarkable opportunity for a modal shift towards active mobility, at least for part of the population and the journeys (De Vos 2020). Specific cycling amenities (which gave rise to the term "*coronapistes*" in French or "pop-up bike lanes") were developed on an experimental basis in record time in many cities in France and around the world (such as Boston, Berlin, Bogotá) in the context of the Covid-19 health-related crisis, in view of promoting cycling and responding to demand.

In its release from lockdown plan, the city of Paris ensured the construction of 50 kilometer temporary additional cycling lanes (out of a total of 1,000 km) from May 2020. 100 km of supplementary lanes were developed in the same way and at the same time in the inner suburbs of the Paris region. Many other French cities (e.g. Lyon, Nantes, Montpellier, Tours, Angers) developed temporary cycling lanes in the context of the health crisis, and the majority of these cities intend to perpetuate all or part of these lanes.

3. These data present the evolution in the frequentation of places such as public transport stations in geographical areas (around the world) based on information from Google users who have activated the "location history" parameter. Data are aggregated and anonymized via the same algorithm used by Google to show the peak times of different places in Google Maps. See: https://www.google.com/covid19/mobility/index.html?hl=en.

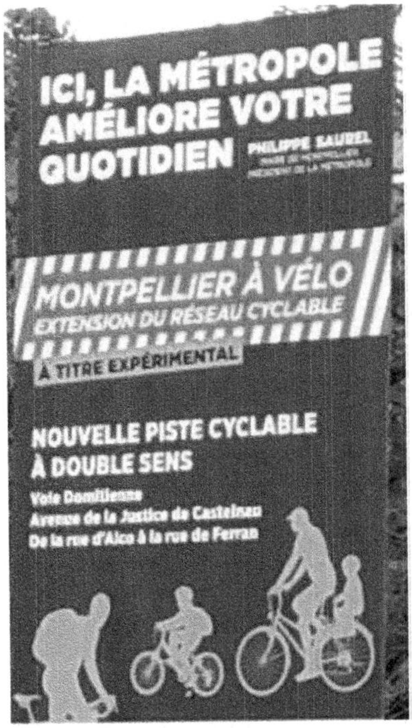
ICI, LA MÉTROPOLE
AMÉLIORE VOTRE
QUOTIDIEN
MONTPELLIER À VÉLO
EXTENSION DU RÉSEAU CYCLABLE
À TITRE EXPÉRIMENTAL
NOUVELLE PISTE CYCLABLE
À DOUBLE SENS

a)

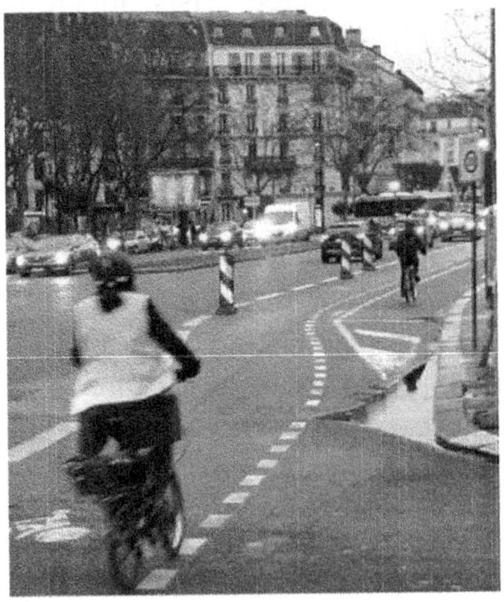

b)

**Figure 5.2.** *a) Development of the experimental cycling network in Montpellier, France (June 2020, H. Charreire). b) Experimental cycling lane between Paris and Saint-Mandé, France (January 2021, H. Charreire). For a color version of this figure, see www.iste.co.uk/vallee/everyday.zip*

This has also made it possible to accelerate pre-existing infrastructure projects, as in the case of the *Réseau express régional vélo d'Île-de-France.* As for public decision-makers and urban planners, the major challenge of the post-Covid-19 transition will be to facilitate a modal transfer of public transport towards active modes, rather than towards the individual car. While evaluations are currently still uncommon, the first results are mixed (Abdullah et al. 2020). In this context of crisis, cities have shown that they are able to deploy equipment in very short time frames. This type of operation can be pursued by inviting the population to co-construct and become involved in the sustainability of cycling and pedestrian amenities.

Tackling Covid-19, (or at least some of its severe forms, which risk evolving unfavorably), means fighting against its main associated comorbidities such as obesity, hypertension, diabetes, cardiovascular and chronic respiratory disorders and cancer. Physical activity is crucial in this fight (Lancet 2020). While it is too early to comment on the underlying mechanisms fueling pandemic deaths, the dangerous relationship between diabetes and Covid-19 has received particular attention (Cariou et al. 2020), as has occurred with the obesity and Covid-19 relationship (Caussy et al. 2020).

## 5.5. Conclusion

The urban environment is one of the major determinants of health-related behaviors, in particular active mobility and in broader terms, physical activity. Therefore, one of the challenges public decision-makers face is to support the transition underway and to favor urban planning designs that promote the health and well-being of all populations, while respecting the Sustainable Development Goals (SDG). These dimensions are the basis of healthy cities, promoted since 1987 by the WHO Healthy Cities program.

The persistence of social and spatial inequalities in health and the awareness of the influence of the living environment on health-related behaviors require us to question the way in which urban planning choices affect physical activity and active mobility practices, especially among the most vulnerable populations.

To meet this challenge, close collaboration between urban planners and public health stakeholders must be formalized around joint reflections on strategies for developing the city, as well as for supporting and encouraging urban planning approaches that enhance health and well-being. The goals are twofold:

– on the one hand, to encourage longitudinal research studying the relationships between environment, mobility and health in their territorial context, to better understand its dynamics and fight against inequalities;

– on the other hand, to develop technical recommendations as operational as possible to enable urban planners to integrate health into urban projects.

As such, the emergence of Health Impact Assessment (HIA) policies in France, and the recent dissemination of guides to support local authorities and planners (ADEME, DGALN, DGS 2020), contribute to this dynamic.

## 5.6. References

Abdullah, M., Dias, C., Muley, D., Shahin, M. (2020). Exploring the impacts of COVID-19 on travel behavior and mode preferences. *Transportation Research Interdisciplinary Perspectives*, 8, 100255.

ADEME, DGALN, DGS (2020). Guide ISadOrA : une démarche d'accompagnement à l'intégration de la Santé dans les Opérations d'Aménagement urbain [Online]. Available at: https://librairie.ademe.fr/urbanisme-et-batiment/263-guide-isadora-une-demarche-d-accompagnement-a-l-integration-de-la-sante-dans-les-operations-d-amenagement-urbain-le.html [Accessed 15 November 2021].

Aldred, R., Woodcock, J., Goodman, A. (2021). Major investment in active travel in outer London: Impacts on travel behaviour, physical activity, and health. *Journal of Transport & Health*, 20, 100958.

Anguelovski, I., Triguero-Mas, M., Connolly, J.J., Kotsila, P., Shokry, G., Pulgar, C.P.D., Garcia-Lamarca, M., Argüelles, L., Mangione, J., Dietz, K. et al. (2020). Gentrification and health in two global cities: A call to identify impacts for socially-vulnerable residents. *Cities & Health*, 4(1), 40–49.

Beck, M.J., Hensher, D.A., Wei, E. (2020). Slowly coming out of COVID-19 restrictions in Australia: Implications for working from home and commuting trips by car and public transport. *Journal of Transport Geography*, 88, 102846.

Bhavsar, N.A., Kumar, M., Richman, L. (2020). Defining gentrification for epidemiologic research: A systematic review. *PLoS ONE*, 15(5), e0233361.

Cariou, B., Hadjadj, S., Wargny, M., Pichelin, M., Al-Salameh, A., Allix, I., Amadou, C., Arnault, G., Baudoux, F., Bauduceau, B. et al. (2020). Phenotypic characteristics and prognosis of inpatients with COVID-19 and diabetes: The CORONADO study. *Diabetologia*, 63(8), 1500–1515.

Caussy, C., Pattou, F., Wallet, F., Simon, C., Chalopin, S., Telliam, C., Mathieu, D., Subtil, F., Frobert, E., Alligier, M. et al. (2020). Prevalence of obesity among adult inpatients with COVID-19 in France. *The Lancet. Diabetes & Endocrinology*, 8(7), 562–564.

CEREMA (2015). La mobilité en transition. *Transflash*, 398 [Online]. Available at: http://www.cerema.fr/fr/centre-ressources/newsletters/transflash/transflash-ndeg-398-juin-2015/mobilite-transition [Accessed 15 November 2021].

Cerin, E., Nathan, A., van Cauwenberg, J., Barnett, D.W., Barnett, A., The Council on Environment and Physical Activity (CEPA) (2017). The neighbourhood physical environment and active travel in older adults: A systematic review and meta-analysis. *International Journal of Behavioral Nutrition and Physical Activity*, 14(1), 15.

Chaix, B., Simon, C., Charreire, H., Thomas, F., Kestens, Y., Karusisi, N., Vallée, J., Oppert, J.-M., Weber, C., Pannier, B. (2014). The environmental correlates of overall and neighborhood based recreational walking (a cross-sectional analysis of the RECORD Study). *International Journal of Behavioral Nutrition and Physical Activity*, 11(1), 20.

Chandrabose, M., Rachele, J.N., Gunn, L., Kavanagh, A., Owen, N., Turrell, G., Giles-Corti, B., Sugiyama, T. (2019). Built environment and cardio-metabolic health: Systematic review and meta-analysis of longitudinal studies. *Obesity Reviews*, 20(1), 41–54.

Charreire, H., Feuillet, T., Roda, C., Mackenbach, J.D., Compernolle, S., Glonti, K., Bardos, H., Le Vaillant, M., Rutter, H., McKee, M. et al. (2016). Self-defined residential neighbourhoods: Size variations and correlates across five European urban regions: Self-defined residential neighbourhoods. *Obesity Reviews*, 17, 9–18.

Chen, D.-R. and Truong, K. (2012). Using multilevel modeling and geographically weighted regression to identify spatial variations in the relationship between place-level disadvantages and obesity in Taiwan. *Applied Geography*, 32(2), 737–745.

Cheng, L., Shi, K., De Vos, J., Cao, M., Witlox, F. (2021). Examining the spatially heterogeneous effects of the built environment on walking among older adults. *Transport Policy*, 100, 21–30.

Clifton, K.J., Livi Smith, A.D., Rodriguez, D. (2007). The development and testing of an audit for the pedestrian environment. *Landscape and Urban Planning*, 80(1), 95–110.

Craig, P., Cooper, C., Gunnell, D., Haw, S., Lawson, K., Macintyre, S., Ogilvie, D., Petticrew, M., Reeves, B., Sutton, M. et al. (2012). Using natural experiments to evaluate population health interventions: New medical research council guidance. *Journal of Epidemiology and Community Health*, 66(12), 1182–1186.

Craig, P., Dieppe, P., Macintyre, S., Michie, S., Nazareth, I., Petticrew, M. (2013). Developing and evaluating complex interventions: The new medical research council guidance. *International Journal of Nursing Studies*, 50(5), 587–592.

Cummins, S., Curtis, S., Diez-Roux, A.V., Macintyre, S. (2007). Understanding and representing "place" in health research: A relational approach. *Social Science & Medicine*, 65(9), 1825–1838.

Day, K., Boarnet, M., Alfonzo, M., Forsyth, A. (2006). The Irvine–Minnesota Inventory to measure built environments: Development. *American Journal of Preventive Medicine*, 30(2), 144–152.

De Vos, J. (2020). The effect of COVID-19 and subsequent social distancing on travel behavior. *Transportation Research Interdisciplinary Perspectives*, 5, 100121.

Dixon, B.N., Ugwoaba, U.A., Brockmann, A.N., Ross, K.M. (2021). Associations between the built environment and dietary intake, physical activity, and obesity: A scoping review of reviews. *Obesity Reviews*, 22(4), e13171.

DRIEA (2019). Favoriser la "marchabilité" : un levier d'actions pour améliorer la santé des Franciliens [Online]. Available at: https://www.iledefrance.ars.sante.fr/favoriser-la-marchabilite-un-levier-dactions-pour-ameliorer-la-sante-des-franciliens [Accessed 14 January 2022].

Elshahat, S., O'Rorke, M., Adlakha, D. (2020). Built environment correlates of physical activity in low- and middle-income countries: A systematic review. *PLoS ONE*, 15(3), e0230454.

Ewing, R. and Cervero, R. (2010). Travel and the built environment. *Journal of the American Planning Association*, 76(3), 265–294.

Faka, A., Chalkias, C., Georgousopoulou, E.N., Tripitsidis, A., Pitsavos, C., Panagiotakos, D.B. (2019). Identifying determinants of obesity in Athens, Greece through global and local statistical models. *Spatial and Spatio-Temporal Epidemiology*, 29, 31–41.

Feuillet, T. (2021). Les effets de contexte en géographie. Des fondements théoriques à la modélisation statistique. PhD Thesis, Université Lyon 3 Jean Moulin, Lyon.

Feuillet, T., Salze, P., Charreire, H., Menai, M., Enaux, C., Perchoux, C., Hess, F., Kesse-Guyot, E., Hercberg, S., Simon, C. et al. (2016). Built environment in local relation with walking: Why here and not there? *Journal of Transport & Health*, 3(4), 500–512.

Feuillet, T., Commenges, H., Menai, M., Salze, P., Perchoux, C., Reuillon, R., Kesse-Guyot E., Enaux, C., Nazare, J.A., Hercberg, S. et al. (2018). A massive geographically weighted regression model of walking-environment relationships. *Journal of Transport Geography*, 68, 118–129.

Feuillet, T., Valette, J.F., Charreire, H., Kesse-Guyot, E., Julia, C., Vernez-Moudon, A., Hercberg, S., Touvier, M., Oppert, J.M. (2020). Influence of the urban context on the relationship between neighbourhood deprivation and obesity. *Social Science & Medicine*, 265, 113537.

Frank, L.D., Schmid, T.L., Sallis, J.F., Chapman, J., Saelens, B.E. (2005). Linking objectively measured physical activity with objectively measured urban form: Findings from SMARTRAQ. *American Journal of Preventive Medicine*, 28(2), 117–125.

Fuller, D., Gauvin, L., Kestens, Y., Daniel, M., Fournier, M., Morency, P., Drouin, L. (2013). Impact evaluation of a public bicycle share program on cycling: A case example of BIXI in Montreal, Quebec. *American Journal of Public Health*, 103(3), e85–e92.

Galster, G.C. (2012). The mechanism(s) of neighbourhood effects: Theory, evidence, and policy implications. In *Neighbourhood Effects Research: New Perspectives*, van Ham, M., Manley, D., Bailey, N., Simpson, L., Maclennan, D. (eds). Springer, Dordrecht, 23–56 [Online]. Available at: https://doi.org/10.1007/978-94-007-2309-2_2 [Accessed 12 January 2021].

Gibbons, J., Barton, M., Brault, E. (2018). Evaluating gentrification's relation to neighborhood and city health. *PLoS ONE*, 13(11), e0207432.

Giles-Corti, B., Vernez-Moudon, A., Reis, R., Turrell, G., Dannenberg, A.L., Badland, H., Foster, S., Lowe, M., Sallis, J.F., Stevenson, M. et al. (2016). City planning and population health: A global challenge. *The Lancet*, 388(10062), 2912–2924.

Gkiotsalitis, K. and Cats, O. (2021). Public transport planning adaption under the COVID-19 pandemic crisis: Literature review of research needs and directions. *Transport Reviews*, 41(3), 374–392.

Grasser, G., van Dyck, D., Titze, S., Stronegger, W.J. (2017). A European perspective on GIS-based walkability and active modes of transport. *European Journal of Public Health*, 27(1), 145–151.

Honey-Rosés, J., Anguelovski, I., Chireh, V.K., Daher, C., Konijnendijk van den Bosch, C., Litt, J.S., Mawani, V., McCall M.K., Orellana, A., Sanchez, U. et al. (2020). The impact of COVID-19 on public space: An early review of the emerging questions – Design, perceptions and inequities. *Cities & Health*, 1–17.

Hosford, K., Winters, M., Gauvin, L., Camden, A., Dubé, A.-S., Friedman, S.M., Fuller, D. (2019). Evaluating the impact of implementing public bicycle share programs on cycling: The international bikeshare impacts on cycling and collisions study (IBICCS). *International Journal of Behavioral Nutrition and Physical Activity*, 16(1), 107.

Hu, S. and Chen, P. (2021). Who left riding transit? Examining socioeconomic disparities in the impact of COVID-19 on ridership. *Transportation Research Part D : Transport and Environment*, 90, 102654.

Izenberg, J.M., Mujahid, M.S., Yen, I.H. (2018). Health in changing neighborhoods: A study of the relationship between gentrification and self-rated health in the state of California. *Health & Place*, 52, 188–195.

James, P., Berrigan, D., Hart, J.E., Aaron Hipp, J., Hoehner, C.M., Kerr, J., Major, J.M., Oka, M., Laden, F. (2014). Effects of buffer size and shape on associations between the built environment and energy balance. *Health & Place*, 27, 162–170.

Kestens, Y., Winters, M., Fuller, D., Bell, S., Berscheid, J., Brondeel, R., Cantinotti, M., Datta, G., Gauvin, L., Gough, M. et al. (2019). INTERACT: A comprehensive approach to assess urban form interventions through natural experiments. *BMC Public Health*, 19(1), 51.

Kim, S., Park, S., Jang, K. (2019). Spatially-varying effects of built environment determinants on walking. *Transportation Research Part A: Policy and Practice*, 123, 188–199.

Kramer, D., Droomers, M., Jongeneel-Grimen, B., Wingen, M., Stronks, K., Kunst, A.E. (2014). The impact of area-based initiatives on physical activity trends in deprived areas: A quasi-experimental evaluation of the Dutch district approach. *International Journal of Behavioral Nutrition and Physical Activity*, 11(1), 36.

Kramer, D., Lakerveld, J., Stronks, K., Kunst, A.E. (2017). Uncovering how urban regeneration programs may stimulate leisure-time walking among adults in deprived areas: A realist review. *International Journal of Health Services*, 47(4), 703–724.

Kwan, M.-P. (2012). The uncertain geographic context problem. *Annals of the Association of American Geographers*, 102(5), 958–968.

Lancet, T. (2020). Global health: Time for radical change? *The Lancet*, 396(10258), 1129.

Leatherdale, S.T. (2019). Natural experiment methodology for research: A review of how different methods can support real-world research. *International Journal of Social Research Methodology*, 22(1), 19–35.

Lee, K.H., Heo, J., Jayaraman, R., Dawson, S. (2019). Proximity to parks and natural areas as an environmental determinant to spatial disparities in obesity prevalence. *Applied Geography*, 112, 102074.

Macintyre, S., Ellaway, A., Cummins, S. (2002). Place effects on health: How can we conceptualise, operationalise and measure them? *Social Science & Medicine*, 55(1), 125–139.

MacMillan, F., George, E.S., Feng, X., Merom, D., Bennie, A., Cook, A., Sanders, T., Dwyer, G., Pang, B., Guagliano, J.M., et al. (2018). Do natural experiments of changes in neighborhood built environment impact physical activity and diet? A systematic review. *International Journal of Environmental Research and Public Health*, 15(2), 217.

Manski, C.F. (1993). Identification of endogenous social effects: The reflection problem. *The Review of Economic Studies*, 60(3), 531–542.

McCormack, G.R. and Shiell, A. (2011). In search of causality: A systematic review of the relationship between the built environment and physical activity among adults. *International Journal of Behavioral Nutrition and Physical Activity*, 8(1), 125.

Ministère de la Transition écologique (2019). Comment les Français se déplacent-ils en 2019 ? Résultats de l'enquête mobilité des personnes [Online]. Available at: https://www.statistiques.developpement-durable.gouv.fr/comment-les-francais-se-deplacent-ils-en-2019-resultats-de-lenquete-mobilite-des-personnes [Accessed 15 November 2021].

Mudway, I.S., Dundas, I., Wood, H.E., Marlin, N., Jamaludin, J.B., Bremner, S.A., Cross, L., Grieve, A., Nanzer, A., Barratt, B. et al. (2019). Impact of London's low emission zone on air quality and children's respiratory health: A sequential annual cross-sectional study. *The Lancet Public Health*, 4(1), e28–e40.

Myers, C.A., Slack, T., Martin, C.K., Broyles, S.T., Heymsfield, S.B. (2015). Regional disparities in obesity prevalence in the United States: A spatial regime analysis. *Obesity*, 23(2), 481–487.

Ogilvie, D., Adams, J., Bauman, A., Gregg, E.W., Panter, J., Siegel, K.R., Wareham, N.J., White, M. (2020). Using natural experimental studies to guide public health action: Turning the evidence-based medicine paradigm on its head. *Journal of Epidemiology and Community Health*, 74(2), 203–208.

Oshan, T.M., Smith, J.P., Fotheringham, A.S. (2020). Targeting the spatial context of obesity determinants via multiscale geographically weighted regression. *International Journal of Health Geographics*, 19(1), 11.

Panter, J., Guell, C., Humphreys, D., Ogilvie, D. (2019). Can changing the physical environment promote walking and cycling? A systematic review of what works and how. *Health & Place*, 58, 102161.

Perchoux, C., Chaix, B., Cummins, S., Kestens, Y. (2013). Conceptualization and measurement of environmental exposure in epidemiology: Accounting for activity space related to daily mobility. *Health & Place*, 21, 86–93.

Perchoux, C., Chaix, B., Kestens, Y. (2019). Activity spaces in place and health research: Novel exposure measures, data collection tools, and designs. *Health & Place*, 58, 102130.

Peters, M., Muellmann, S., Christianson, L., Stalling, I., Bammann, K., Drell, C., Forberger, S. (2020). Measuring the association of objective and perceived neighborhood environment with physical activity in older adults: Challenges and implications from a systematic review. *International Journal of Health Geographics*, 19(1), 47.

Petrović, A., Manley, D., van Ham, M. (2020). Freedom from the tyranny of neighbourhood: Rethinking sociospatial context effects. *Progress in Human Geography*, 44(6), 1103–1123.

Petticrew, M. (2011). When are complex interventions "complex"? When are simple interventions "simple"? *European Journal of Public Health*, 21(4), 397–398.

Pullano, G., Valdano, E., Scarpa, N., Rubrichi, S., Colizza, V. (2020). Evaluating the effect of demographic factors, socioeconomic factors, and risk aversion on mobility during the COVID-19 epidemic in France under lockdown: A population-based study. *The Lancet Digital Health*, 2(12), e638–e649.

Raulin, F., Lord, S., Negron-Poblete, P. (2016). Évaluation de la marchabilité de trois environnements urbains de la région métropolitaine montréalaise à partir de l'outil MAPPA. *eVertigO, la revue électronique en sciences de l'environnement* [Online]. Available at: https://journals.openedition.org/vertigo/17774 [Accessed 14 January 2022].

Saelens, B.E. and Handy, S.L. (2008). Built environment correlates of walking: A review. *Medicine and Science in Sports and Exercise*, 40(7 Suppl), S550–S566.

Sallis, J.F. and Glanz, K. (2006). The role of built environments in physical activity, eating, and obesity in childhood. *The Future of Children*, 16(1), 89–108.

Sallis, J.F., Floyd, M.F., Rodríguez, D.A., Saelens, B.E. (2012). Role of built environments in physical activity, obesity, and cardiovascular disease. *Circulation*, 125(5), 729–737.

Sallis, J.F., Cerin, E., Kerr, J., Adams, M.A., Sugiyama, T., Christiansen, L.B., Schipperijn, J., Davey, R., Salvo, D., Frank, L.D. et al. (2020). Built environment, physical activity, and obesity: Findings from the International Physical Activity and Environment Network (IPEN) adult study. *Annual Review of Public Health*, 41(1), 119–139.

Santé Publique France (2017). Étude de santé sur l'environnement, la biosurveillance, l'activité physique et la nutrition (Esteban), 2014–2016 [Online]. Available at: https://www.santepubliquefrance.fr/determinants-de-sante/nutrition-et-activite-physique/etude-de-sante-sur-l-environnement-la-biosurveillance-l-activite-physique-et-la-nutrition-esteban-2014-2016.-volet-nutrition.-chapitre-corpulence [Accessed 15 November 2021].

Strominger, J., Anthopolos, R., Miranda, M.L. (2016). Implications of construction method and spatial scale on measures of the built environment. *International Journal of Health Geographics*, 15(1), 15.

Tharrey, M. (2020). Impact de la participation à un jardin partagé en ville sur l'adoption de styles de vie plus durables. PhD Thesis, SupAgro, Montpellier [Online]. Available at: http://www.theses.fr/s184705 [Accessed 25 January 2021].

Tharrey, M., Perignon, M., Scheromm, P., Mejean, C., Darmon, N. (2019). Does participating in community gardens promote sustainable lifestyles in urban settings? Design and protocol of the JArDinS study. *BMC Public Health*, 19(1), 589.

Tirachini, A. and Cats, O. (2020). COVID-19 and public transportation: Current assessment, prospects, and research needs. *Journal of Public Transportation*, 22(1) [Online]. Available at: https://scholarcommons.usf.edu/jpt/vol22/iss1/1.

Vallée, J. (2017). The daycourse of place. *Social Science & Medicine*, 194, 177–181.

Vallée, J., Le Roux, G., Chaix, B., Kestens, Y., Chauvin, P. (2015). The "constant size neighbourhood trap" in accessibility and health studies. *Urban Studies*, 52(2), 338–357.

Van Cauwenberg, J., Clarys, P., De Bourdeaudhuij, I., Van Holle, V., Verté, D., De Witte, N., De Donder, L., Buffel, T., Dury, S., Deforche, B. (2012). Physical environmental factors related to walking and cycling in older adults: The Belgian aging studies. *BMC Public Health*, 12(1), 142.

Van Holle, V., Deforche, B., Van Cauwenberg, J., Goubert, L., Maes, L., Van de Weghe, N., De Bourdeaudhuij, I. (2012). Relationship between the physical environment and different domains of physical activity in European adults: A systematic review. *BMC Public Health*, 12(1), 807.

Van Holle, V., Van Cauwenberg, J., Van Dyck, D., Deforche, B., Van de Weghe, N., De Bourdeaudhuij, I. (2014). Relationship between neighborhood walkability and older adults' physical activity: Results from the Belgian Environmental Physical Activity Study in Seniors (BEPAS Seniors). *International Journal of Behavioral Nutrition and Physical Activity*, 11(1), 110.

Wen, T.-H., Chen, D.-R., Tsai, M.-J. (2010). Identifying geographical variations in poverty-obesity relationships: Empirical evidence from Taiwan. *Geospatial Health*, 4(2), 257–265.

Yang, Y., Wu, X., Zhou, P., Gou, Z., Lu, Y. (2019). Towards a cycling-friendly city: An updated review of the associations between built environment and cycling behaviors (2007–2017). *Journal of Transport & Health*, 14, 100613.

# PART 3

# Daily Mobility and Public Health Policies

# 6

# A Critical Analysis of Policies Promoting Physical Activity and Active Mobility

**Stephanie ALEXANDER**
*Fondation d'entreprise MGEN, pour la santé publique, Paris, France*

## 6.1. Introduction

Daily mobility is a multi-faceted concept, but it mainly refers to "active mobility", the active movement of the body involving an energy consumption exceeding its minimum daily expenditure. "Active mobility" is at the heart of prevention and physical activity promotion campaigns, launched by public health authorities (WHO French Healthy Cities Network 2013).

In the literature, the terms "active mobility" and "physical activity" are often used interchangeably, although the term physical activity implies less of a connection to the physical and social environment, while "active mobility" points to movement through space, which is not always the case for "physical activity". For example, we may speak of "physical activity" independently of the environment surrounding individuals, even though it is often this environment – together with its possibilities and constraints – that encourages or hinders the practice of "physical activity". As such, if we consider that the environment plays an important role in "physical activity", using the term "active mobility" would be more appropriate. However, given the fact that most public health documents use the term "physical activity" when referring to "active mobility", the term "physical activity" will be chosen in this chapter whenever it is used in the document under discussion.

According to the daily active mobility report from the WHO French Healthy Cities Network (*Réseau français des Villes-Santé de l'OMS*) (2013, p. 14), active mobility is defined by "modes of travel such as walking, cycling or rollerblading" that are alternatives to motorized travel. This mode of travel does not generate polluting emissions and, most importantly, it promotes physical activity. The benefits of "active mobility" that are most often mentioned by public health authorities include: a reduction in the risk of chronic disease (diabetes, hypertension, dyslipidemia, cancer, rheumatism) as well as better mental health (reduction in stress, anxiety and depression, self-esteem and physical skills) and physical health (weight maintenance and muscle mass development) (Thibault et al. 2008; Rostan et al. 2011; WHO French Healthy Cities Network 2013; Praznoczy et al. 2017). Active mobility is most often associated with a reduction in premature mortality (WHO French Healthy Cities Network 2013).

The economic cost of a sedentary population for the health system is often brought forward to justify the importance of public health policies promoting active mobility. The report from the *Institut national de prévention et d'éducation pour la santé* (INPES, French National Institute for Prevention and Health Education) (Rostan et al. 2011) states that the "the cost of physical inactivity for the health system has not been accurately assessed in France" (Ibid. 2011, p. 23), whereas in Canada "the estimates show that a less active person might spend 38% more days in hospital, consult their general practitioner 5.5% more often and a medical specialist 13% more often than an active individual" (Ibid. 2011, p. 23). The WHO French Healthy Cities Network report (2013) states that "the proportion of the overall healthcare cost in France attributable to physical inactivity amounts to 2.5%". Finally, according to the *Institut national de la santé et de la recherche médicale* (INSERM, French National Institute of Health and Medical Research 2008, p. 14), "more physical activity on a daily basis can contribute to saving 2 billion euros on diabetes care, 2.2 billion euros on obesity-related expenditures, and a reduction of 500 million euros on the treatment of cholesterol".

While the benefits of active mobility are undeniable for the physical and psychological health of adults, they are particularly important for children and adolescents, producing not only an immediate impact, but also long-lasting effects. According to the authors of the report "Promoting physical activity among young people: designing and developing an Icaps-type project" (Rostan et al. 2011), when the youth take pleasure in physical activities (regardless of the activity's degree of intensity), the benefits of the physical activity extend well into adulthood (Rostan et al. 2011). Active mobility also promotes cohesion and social integration when it takes place in public spaces accessible to a diverse population, such as, for instance, children's streets (United Nations Children's Fund 2012).

Given the work highlighting the benefits of active mobility, public health institutions strongly encourage physical activity and active mobility for adults and children, via general recommendations and health campaigns. These campaigns are increasing in number to prevent an increase in sedentary lifestyles and to promote the social, psychological and physical benefits of daily physical activity (Institut national de la santé et de la recherche médicale (INSERM) 2008; WHO French Healthy Cities Network 2013; Active Healthy Kids Global Alliance 2020; Lemonnier et al. 2020; ONAPS 2020).

All of these physical activity recommendations and campaigns share the goal of preventing disease and promoting healthy living, and they also have in common another element: implicit assumptions and values about the population's health and well-being. However, these assumptions and values may have unexpected effects on the population, which are rarely discussed. This chapter examines these implicit assumptions and values underlying public health policies. By introducing recommendations for promoting physical activity, this chapter aims to analyze and understand their possible unexpected effects, beyond health-related questions in the strictest sense. The analytical approach developed by political scientist Carol Bacchi is given particular attention (Bacchi 2009; Bletsas and Beasley 2012). The critical analysis approach developed by Bacchi (2009) does not imply rejecting public health policies or recommendations, but rather aims to bring to light the implicit assumptions underlying them. In doing so, it is possible to discuss their potentially negative effects in order to improve recommendations and prevent an increase in social inequalities in health.

This chapter begins by outlining the historical context of international recommendations for physical activity and active mobility and then describes the development of policies and actions in Canada and France. Some of these policies and actions are finally discussed from the perspective of Carol Bacchi's (2009) analytical approach.

## 6.2. Historical context of recommendations for daily physical activity

Since at least the 1970s, consensus has developed among international scientists on the importance of practicing physical activity on a daily basis, and this not only for athletes but for the whole population (Favier-Ambrosini 2016). It was the overall decrease in physical activity and the increase in sedentary behavior observed since the 1970s (Cavill et al. 2006) as well as accompanying health disorders (such as obesity, muscular problems and cardiovascular problems) that generated awareness of the importance of physical activity in North America and Europe. This gave birth to a dynamic aimed at encouraging the general population to be more active (Thibault et al. 2008; World Health Organization and Commission on Ending Childhood Obesity 2016; World Health Organization 2018; Active Healthy Kids Global Alliance 2020; Lemonnier et al. 2020; ONAPS 2020). During the 1970s, some health experts began to develop measures to systematically compare the effect of different levels of physical activity on health and to set up specific recommendations regarding the physical activities to be practiced (Centers for Disease Control and Prevention 1996).

The first recommendations mainly targeted cardiorespiratory health and body composition (Centers for Disease Control and Prevention 1996). In an initial report published in 1978, "The recommended quantity and quality of exercise for developing and maintaining fitness in healthy adults" (1996), the frequency and duration of physical activity recommended for all adults were: physical activity three to five times per week, with a 60–90% heart rate increase during 15–60 minutes of activities such as walking, running, cycling, etc. (Centers for Disease Control and Prevention 1996). This report was the basis for the recommendations made well until the 1990s, even though the frequency and intensity of the recommended physical activity proved difficult to follow for the whole population.

The measures and thresholds for physical activity changed over time and recommendations for the frequency, intensity and duration of physical activity were rewritten several times (Centers for Disease Control and Prevention 1996). As of the 1990s, the benefits of more moderate forms of physical activity and alternative types of physical activity were progressively brought forward, giving rise to the publication of a second report taking into account older people and those with reduced mobility. This second report suggested that health benefits could also be appreciated at more moderate intensities than previously believed. Indeed, some studies have shown that there are "dose–response" gradients between the level of physical activity and its positive effect on health (Centers for Disease Control and Prevention 1996). The recommendations for various types of populations were adapted accordingly (older people, people with cardiovascular diseases, etc.), through the calculation of the precise number of minutes of physical activity to be done per day at a certain intensity (Centers for Disease Control and Prevention 1996).

Currently, the thresholds generally accepted as "good health" indicators for adults and children are: 30–60 minutes of moderate physical activity most days, either in a single session or divided into shorter sessions (8–10 minutes) (World Health Organization 2010). With these more flexible measures, the report recognized that people who cannot, or who are not keen to engage in vigorous physical activity can also draw substantial benefit from moderate-intensity physical activity (Centers for Disease Control and Prevention 1996; World Health Organization, Europe 2015; World Health Organization 2020). Over the past few decades, recommendations have evolved, which proves the contingent nature of knowledge (and measures) concerning physical activity and health.

## 6.3. Policies and actions to promote physical activity in Canada and France

### 6.3.1. *The development of policies and actions in Canada*

In 1997, in Canada, while physical activity recommendations were being discussed at the international level, the federal-provincial and territorial ministries in charge of sport, physical activity and recreation had also approved the development of a Canadian guide to combat the increasing physical inactivity observed in the country (Sharratt and Hearst 2007). Developed over one year, researchers specializing in physical activity and sport worked on Canada's first physical activity guide (*Canada's Physical Activity Guide to Healthy Active Living*), which was published in 1998 by Health Canada and the Canadian Society for Exercise Physiology (CSEP) (Sharratt and Hearst 2007). This first guide was based on Canadian research conducted by members from the CSEP and on international guides about physical activity (Sharratt and Hearst 2007). It introduced up-to-date recommendations in order to promote physical activity among adults in Canada (18–55 years old). The guide was useful for accurately evaluating the population's level of physical activity. A year later, in 1999, a second guide was developed, suitable for adults aged 55 and over (Sharratt and Hearst 2007). Given the scope of the discussions around "the childhood obesity epidemic" (Moffat 2010) in the 1990s, and the urgent calls from public health institutions, doctors and professionals working on childhood health to fight the epidemic, three new CSEP physical activity guides were developed: one for children aged 5–9 years, one for young people aged 10–17 years (Sharratt and Hearst 2007; Tremblay et al. 2012, 2014), and the latest issue promoting physical activity for babies and children between 0 and 4 years old (Canadian Society for Exercise Physiology 2020).

The physical activity recommendations presented in the CSEP guides were subsequently taken up by other Canadian organizations. For example, ParticipAction, an organization created in the 1970s and funded by the Canadian government in response to scientific findings, had already signaled the risk of low physical activity among Canadians (Bauman et al. 2004; Edwards 2004). Despite the transformations of the organization since the 1970s, ParticipAction is known for having conducted physical activity promotion campaigns throughout the years, often with humor and creativity, to encourage Canadians to move more, namely through simple daily activities (cleaning, playing, active transportation, etc.). ParticipAction has launched numerous campaigns to promote physical activity since 1997, based on the recommendations published in the CSEP guides, according to different age groups. Since 2007, the organization has mainly targeted physical activity for young people and has become the main voice for communicating the importance of physical activity and active mobility among young people (Canadian Society for Exercise Physiology 2011).

Active Healthy Kids Canada is another Canadian organization that evaluates and promotes physical activity for young people. After the strong advocacy of the Canadian government to promote physical activity among young people and combat "the childhood obesity epidemic", a panel of experts met in 2004 to discuss and develop the most relevant indicators for evaluating physical activity among young Canadians and taking better action. This meeting was the basis for the "Canadian Report Cards on Physical Activity for Children and Youth" (hereafter referred to as report cards), which have been published almost annually since 2005 (Active Healthy Kids Canada 2005). The report cards aim to assess different facets of physical activity and areas of influence on physical activity among the youth (Active Healthy Kids Canada 2005). From the outset, the publication of the report cards was based on the guidelines and recommendations made by the CSEP to provide physical activity assessment for young people.

Physical activity indicators, created by researchers and members of the Active Healthy Kids Canada organization in charge of developing the report cards, included three main categories:

– individual behavior (overall physical activity, participation in organized sport, active play, active transport/mobility, sedentary behavior);

– spheres of influence on physical activity (family and peers, school, community and the built environment);

– government and non-government strategies and investments (Active Healthy Kids Canada 2005; Tremblay et al. 2014).

The purpose of the report cards is to assess these indicators and award them a grade (A, B, C, D, etc.). According to the ratings assigned to them, these three main categories are evaluated every year to determine the progress of political strategies, the different spheres of influence and the population's behavior in terms of physical activity. Results are expressed in the form of simple "grades", designed as a communication tool to inform the public and public health organizations, to create better health policies and to stimulate social action by encouraging debate (Tremblay et al. 2014). Each report card provides valuable information on whether overall physical activity categories meet expectations and which are to be improved, issuing action recommendations for each of these categories (Tremblay et al. 2014). With the publication of report cards, Active Healthy Kids Canada also hoped to encourage the government to fund new programs and to create policies and concrete actions promoting physical activity among young people. Since 2015, report cards have been produced and published by the organization ParticipAction, always with the mission of promoting physical activity and active mobility among the youth based on evaluation indicators and advocating for the changes to be made in the various spheres of influence (public policies, transport, school, family, individual behavior, etc.).

### 6.3.2. *The development of policies and actions in France*

In France, the promotion of physical activity and its explicit integration into public health policies emerged in the early 2000s with the publication of the first French National Nutrition and Health Program (PNNS, *Programme national nutrition santé*) in 2001 (Prévot-Ledrich et al. 2016; Vuillemin

2018). The PNNS issues dietary and physical activity recommendations for adults, pregnant women, people over 55, children and adolescents (French Ministry of Solidarity and Health 2019). Among other objectives, the most recent PNNS from 2019 includes the objective "of encouraging active mobility", by means of two specific actions:

– promoting local interventions making physical activity an easy, pleasant, secure practice;

– favoring active mobility for daily transportation (French Ministry of Solidarity and Health 2019, pp. 32–33).

Various activities have been proposed to match these actions, such as the development of walking buses or biking buses for school transportation, the development of playgrounds and the integration of green spaces and recreational facilities in urban planning (2019, pp. 32–33). The "Cycling Plan" (*Plan Vélo*) and the development of cycling amenities are also mentioned as a means of promoting active mobility.

The first National Nutrition and Health Program and subsequent editions initiated a dynamic for promoting physical activity in France, which was taken up by several organizations. In 2013, the WHO French Healthy Cities Network published a practical action guide placing active mobility at the center of their recommendations: "Daily active mobility: the role of communities" (WHO French Healthy Cities Network 2013). With this guide, the actors involved aimed to facilitate the implementation of local policies in favor of active mobility and to promote daily physical activity in the population (WHO French Healthy Cities Network 2013).

In 2015, the French National Observatory of Physical Activity and Sedentary Behaviors (*Observatoire National de l'Activité Physique et de la Sédentarité*) (ONAPS) was created on the initiative of the Ministry in charge of sports and the National Center for Sport Development. Its purpose was to develop a scientific approach to measure the impact of physical activity and sedentariness on the health of the French population (ONAPS 2021). A year later, working with the key members behind the Canadian physical activity report cards and by following their model and its methodology, the members of ONAPS and researchers working in the field of sport and physical activity developed and published the first physical activity report card for France, entitled "Physical activity and sedentariness in children and adolescents: First inventory in France" (ONAPS 2016). According to the authors, the 2016 French report card was an opportunity to highlight the environmental, institutional and family levers of physical activity among the youth. Since 2016, ONAPS has produced two other report cards (2018 and 2020) with the goal of evaluating the progression of physical activity among the French youth, making recommendations to increase physical activity and identifying intersectoral actions to improve the health of young people through physical activity.

This new dynamic around physical activity was also supported by the strategy adopted by the WHO Europe (2015), which encourages European countries to integrate physical activity recommendations into their public policies (Prévot-Ledrich et al. 2016). In 2018, a tool was developed in France to facilitate the implementation of physical activity actions: the CAPLA-Santé (*Cadre d'analyse des politiques locales activité physique – Santé*) (Noël Racine et al. 2021). This tool was an adaptation of the WHO public policy analysis tool (the HEPA, Health Enhancing Physical Activity) by a multi-disciplinary panel of intersectoral experts. It was intended for all the territorial communities and their partners to assist in intersectoral work and to advocate for the development and implementation of physical activity policies (Cambon et al. 2021). It allows for the analysis of policies and their contexts in order to measure the progress made in physical activity and health promotion, intersectoral collaboration and the identification of effective policy levers (Noël Racine et al. 2021).

As such, physical activity was at the heart of public health intervention programs and strategies in France. In 2020, *Santé publique France*[1] published the issue "Promoting health through sports and physical activity" (Lemonnier et al. 2020), which discusses the roles that sports clubs, communities and the everyday places in which we live can play in promoting better health (Lemonnier et al. 2020). The issue suggested a "change of paradigm: shifting from a care logic to a preventive logic […] to promote physical activity from an early age and, more broadly, to develop the individual and collective health capital of all French citizens […] by adapting the environment" (Ibid. p. 3). For the authors, this involved adopting an "intersectoral" approach to health, associating the environment, modes of transportation, design of the city or the territory, the challenges of

1. *Santé publique France* is the national public health agency in France, whose mission is to improve and protect the health of the population.

urban planning and the motivations and behavior of the population living there. An example of this intersectoral approach is the "*Plan Vélo et mobilités actives*" ("Cycling and active mobility plan"), implemented by the French Ministry of Ecological Transition in 2018, aiming to render cycling a real mode of transportation for the population (French Ministry of Ecological Transition 2019). The *Plan vélo et mobilités actives* states that:

> Being non-polluting, inexpensive, accessible to all and good for health, cycling has many benefits for users and the community. France should place this mode of transportation at the heart of mobility considerations. The plan proposed by the Government aims to triple the use of bicycles … (Ibid. p. 6).

To conclude this section focusing on the policies and actions carried out in Canada and France, we can highlight the growing desire in both countries to create living environments and policies conducive to physical activity and active mobility, as well as to make the recent knowledge about them accessible to actors from different backgrounds. The two countries also share an interest in promoting physical activity among the youth by means of physical activity report cards. These report cards have become an innovative way for researchers in the field of physical activity and organizations dedicated to the promotion of physical activity to begin to address this need, in particular by developing a rigorous and common methodology for collecting evidence on physical activity among young people and communicating practical recommendations for action.

In 2014, in response to instigation by the World Health Organization (WHO) to take action against the childhood obesity epidemic at a global scale, the organization Active Healthy Kids (developers of the report cards) created Active Healthy Kids Global Alliance (2020). The goals of the Global Alliance included bringing together researchers and organizations around the world on the subject of physical activity for young people, disseminating the report card methodology for the creation and evaluation of indicators and working with international researchers so that they could also publish a physical activity report card in their countries. In 2016, there were already 38 member countries adhering to the Global Alliance, including France (Aubert et al. 2019; Active Healthy Kids Global Alliance 2020), all of whom were committed to developing and measuring physical activity indicators and creating report cards in their countries (Aubert et al. 2019).

## 6.4. The implicit values underlying policies promoting physical activity and active mobility: what questions should be asked?

Organizations recommending physical activity share the goal of preventing disease and promoting a healthy lifestyle for the population. Measures have been developed to identify where and at which population physical activity recommendations can be targeted. As mentioned in the introduction of this chapter, these recommendations often include implicit assumptions and values about the population's health and well-being. The question-posing approach developed by political scientist Carol Bacchi in her book *Analyzing Policy: What's the problem represented to be?* (Bacchi 2009; Bletsas and Beasley 2012) helps to uncover these assumptions and values to better understand why a certain policy or intervention may have a greater or lesser impact on a given group or population. Bacchi's (2009) approach includes an analytical guide drawing on the writings of Michel Foucault (Foucault 1997; Bacchi 2010) and his discussions on "problematizations". This guide helps to analyze the thoughts underlying certain forms of governance or policies: it is useful not only for challenging assumptions that have been taken for granted in institutional documents and policies (Bacchi 2009, p. 30) but also for explaining the way in which certain public health problems are thought of and written about, as well as the solutions proposed.

In this chapter, Bacchi's question-posing approach will be used as an analytical tool for detecting the possible "blind spots" in policies promoting physical activity and active mobility. This approach does not intend to reject public health recommendations, but rather seeks to highlight the (potentially negative) effects of certain recommendations and identify why certain interventions have failed, in order to improve them and prevent an increase in social inequalities in health. Three sets of questions adapted from Bacchi's "question-posing approach" (2009) will be used as a common thread.

### 6.4.1. *What is the "problem" represented to be in the policies promoting physical activity and active mobility?*

Institutional and political discourses dictate the dominant representations of the "problems" that require intervention. In this sense, a first step is to call into question the assumption that governing political actors are simply reacting to problems that already exist "out in the world", an idea that

Bacchi (2009) considers to be taken for granted. Bacchi (2009) has argued that the dominant representations of a problem only reflect one of the many possible alternative constructions of a given problem. For example, a higher body weight can be interpreted either as a health risk or as a sign of well-being and good nutrition, depending on the place and time being considered. Despite this, given the fact that governments and public health institutions occupy a privileged position, it is their construction and understanding of contemporary issues that prevail and are addressed by public policies and interventions (Bacchi 2009). These ways of constructing and representing problems deserve to be carefully examined.

The question posed at the beginning of this section encourages us to explicitly describe the issues these interventions seek to respond to. To begin with, the identification of the solutions suggested for problems reveals the way the problem has been understood and perceived. This can be useful for dissecting the representation of the problem. Indeed, often the problem – as represented in the documents – is only one of multiple representations of the problem. Take, for example, the promotion of physical activity among young children. The report cards focus on programs that promote "active play" for children in order to change the way they play. By analyzing the texts that recommend increasing children's active play – while putting aside sedentary play – we can identify the underlying problem represented in the documents: they assume that children do not play in the right way – or rather, not in a sufficiently healthy way.

The recommended solutions are visible through the nine main indicators on report cards, among which is the "active play" indicator. This indicator was created and added to the Canadian report cards in 2008 and has appeared in all report cards developed by the Global Alliance member countries since 2014, including the French ones (2018–2020). The most striking fact is that the "active play" indicator has systematically been included as one of the nine main indicators on report cards, despite often being described as "inconclusive" or as relying on "insufficient data", and rarely being awarded a grade. The fact that an indicator that cannot be measured or graded is maintained as one of the nine central report card indicators demonstrates the interest and commitment that researchers have in the notion of children's "active play", and the institutional claim that "active play" is an essential activity for promoting child well-being. This commitment is at the origin of the solutions proposed by institutions and organizations in order to modify children's leisure activities by limiting sedentary play and increasing active play.

### 6.4.2. *What concepts/categories, knowledge and values underlie these recommendations? Who is excluded from these discourses?*

According to Bacchi (2009), it does not suffice to analyze the way in which problems are represented and the solutions recommended. It is necessary to go further and identify the concepts, categories and knowledge engaged to describe the world, define the population targeted and create interventions. These concepts, categories and knowledge are often taken for granted and rarely called into question. By examining the way in which they are used in discourses, we can begin to identify the values and priorities on which they – and subsequently the interventions – are based. The goal of this chapter is not to call into question the values of individuals, nor those of the organizations responsible for developing interventions, but rather to render explicit the social and cultural values and priorities rooted in collective thought. In doing so, the aim here is to shed light on a kind of "social unconscious" (Bacchi 2009), which underlies the policies promoting physical activity and active mobility.

First, the concepts and categories chosen to characterize people (the young, the elderly, the homeless, the sick, obese people, etc.) should be carefully identified and examined, because they are based on values and priorities that are not universal; categories and concepts often have a specific history (Bletsas and Beasley 2012).

However, making them explicit is not an easy task because we are all immersed in these social universes and share these historical moments. For example, the concept of "good health" or the category of "obese person" both carry social and cultural values associated with a normative corpulence (a maximum body size defined as "good health"), with specific lifestyle habits (desired activities and behaviors) and with the rejection of excess (certain foods, smoking, alcohol, etc.).

While the values inherent in the concept of "good health" or the category of "obese person" are often supported and informed by scientific research, they are not only informed by scientific studies, but also by normative values that are not relevant for all populations nor for all the members of the same population. For example, in relation to the concept of "good health", being underweight (BMI[2] lower than 18.5) is less likely to be defined as unhealthy than being overweight (BMI between 25 and 30), despite some studies having shown that there is excess mortality associated with being underweight, but not for being overweight (Flegal 2005; Flegal et al. 2007; Veronese et al. 2015; Egom et al. 2018). For some populations, especially older people, being slightly overweight can even be protective against certain diseases (Veronese et al. 2015).

Furthermore, being in "good health", outwardly expressed by a toned body and by a person who engages in physical activity, is sometimes considered to be equivalent to a kind of morality (LeBesco 2011). In this example, a normative physical appearance is prioritized, one that represents "good health", yet without a health status necessarily being correlated to it. The category of "obese person", often used as a definition of the person instead of simply describing a state, is also problematic. It attaches social and cultural values to the person (deemed unhealthy, having bad lifestyle habits, suffering from a lack of motivation to do physical activity, lazy, leading a life of excess, etc.). In addition, obesity is defined by a BMI whose relevance and accuracy are strongly debated and does not apply equally to all populations (Humphreys 2010; Egom et al. 2018; Gutin 2018; The Lancet Gastroenterology and Hepatology 2019).

Second, we can also question the knowledge at the heart of physical activity interventions, which predominantly adopts a biomedical view of human health (Gard and Wright 2001; Etkin 2016); an implicit value in public health more broadly. For example, the first measurements and recommendations related to physical activity and sport were based on quantitative indicators (30–60 minutes of physical activity, three to five times a week) and biomedical measurements (heart rate, % muscle, % fat) (Gard and Wright 2001; Etkin 2016). The promotion of the "biomedical" approach and the priority given to quantitative measurements explain why the recommendations often neglect non-biomedical aspects of physical activities (sensations, psychological effort, well-being during the activity, perception of one's own body, etc.). These non-biomedical aspects have been discussed less, because they are less valued despite also being important for the practice of physical activity, in particular for understanding motivation and pleasure, or dislike of physical activity (Adams 2019). The number of minutes spent engaging in a physical activity reveals nothing

2. BMI is the abbreviation for "Body Mass Index", calculated by dividing weight (in kg) by the height's square (in m).

about the well-being of the person who is practicing the activity, nor about the overall benefit such activity may bring. Recommendations for physical activity mainly focus their attention on improving physical health while neglecting the improvement of the person's overall well-being (Alexander et al. 2014a).

Third, the values underlying public health policies ought to be analyzed, regardless of whether they are values anchored in these policies or those excluded from mainstream discussions (or less promoted ones). As noted earlier, interventions promoting physical activity and active mobility prioritize improving physical health (through physical activity), often neglecting the notion of pleasure. For example, in the report cards, as in many interventions, sedentary activities – especially time spent in front of screens – are presented as dangerous and as posing health risks to young people. While a predominantly sedentary lifestyle can certainly pose physical health problems (loss of muscles, back pain, etc.) (Cavill et al. 2006), demonizing screen time and prescribing physical activity (60 minutes a day) at all costs neglects the element of pleasure in these activities, although it is particularly important especially for children's activities (Alexander et al. 2014b). If physical activity is always promoted with a view to achieving a given result (reducing obesity, promoting ideal health, 150 minutes of weekly physical activity), physical activity risks becoming a simple instrument to achieve a (more or less interesting) goal, rather than an activity that has an intrinsic value (Alexander et al. 2019). Indeed, if physical activity becomes a task or obligation, it is more difficult to maintain the element of pleasure in it (Alexander et al. 2019). Furthermore, if sedentary activities become a symbol of a health risk or hazard which should be avoided at all costs, this may remove the enjoyment that some children derive from quiet and restful sedentary activities, such as reading or making a puzzle (Alexander et al. 2014b).

Finally, the supposedly universal scope of the benefits of an active lifestyle also ought to be revisited and reconsidered according to the values and capabilities of different individuals. Recommendations that promote a culture of physical activity and healthy lifestyle, as well as the policies seeking to "change the paradigm" to "encourage the practice of physical activity from an early age" (*Plan vélo et mobilités actives*), aim to change the population's mentality: they encourage the population to prioritize active forms of mobility and accept the idea that being active is the easiest choice to make. This is undoubtedly good for the majority of the population.

However, the discourses inherent in physical activity and active mobility policies assume that the policies will have a similar or equivalent benefit for everyone in the population. This assumption has to be critically examined because it does not take into account the different types of mobility within the population. Indeed, not all individuals are active in the same way: the benefit that individuals may derive from physical activity depends on the possibility for mobility within the environment in which they live, which may be poorly adapted – not readily accessible – for those who use different modes of transportation (wheelchair, using a guide dog, people who can only move on flat surfaces, etc.). By assuming that physical activity and active mobility benefit everyone equally, these policies overlook the fact that some people cannot increase their level of physical activity and that others may not want to. Although staying active is a public health value, this value is not necessarily a priority for all individuals.

### 6.4.3. *Which populations are targeted by policies and which are excluded?*

The third and last set of questions proposed by Bacchi (2009) focus on the populations targeted and those excluded by the interventions. The intention is to bring to light the unexpected (even negative) effects that public health policies may bring about.

To start with a very common example, we can consider a population frequently targeted by public health policies, that of "obese" people, for which the problem is implicitly represented as being an individual problem. Conceiving obesity as a problem of individual responsibility leads to solutions aimed at the individual alone: a change in diet, an increase in physical activity or other forms of weight management. Even though these recommendations seem obvious and can benefit some individuals, representing the problem mainly as the result of individual actions is problematic because it overlooks the historical, social, contextual and environmental constraints for the individuals concerned (Haut conseil de la santé publique 2018). As such, recommendations such as these can be ineffective or even become a means of exclusion or marginalization for certain populations.

Similarly, recommendations encouraging the population to be active "60 minutes a day" are not suitable for everyone. For example, there are people who would like to be more active, but find it difficult because they have health problems, or some physical impairments, or live in a neighborhood without the space for practicing physical activities (without parks, near streets packed with cars, etc.). The 2016 French report card recommended that policies take into account the multiple factors influencing the physical activity of young people, with "special attention [being] given to children with disabilities or suffering from chronic illnesses, in order to facilitate their access to practice". In order for this recommendation of personal specificities not to be ignored, it is necessary for urban, educational and institutional policies to implement concrete actions. If this is not the case, it will be the people who are already active (members of a sports club, for example) or those potentially active (e.g. residents of neighborhoods in which sports and recreational facilities are numerous and of good quality) who will more easily follow the recommendations for physical activity. On the contrary, people who are not immersed in a favorable context for physical activity will not have the same opportunities to follow those recommendations. Indeed, promoting regular physical activity can widen inequalities between populations (Alexander and Shareck 2021) (see Chapter 3).

As Bacchi (2009) has suggested, the exclusion of certain populations should also be analyzed. Certain exclusions appear in discourses promoting walking and cycling. For example, the *Plan vélo et mobilités actives* ("Cycling and active mobility plan") implemented in France in 2018 by the Ministry of Ecological Transition pointed out that cycling in a calm and peaceful environment can not only lead to an increase in active mobility and a reduction in environmental pollution (atmospheric pollution, noise, etc.), but can also contribute to greater mental well-being (French Ministry of Ecological Transition 2019). This position, which is at the origin of policies aimed at promoting health in a global way (physical, social and mental health), assumes that the entire population has access to calm environments suitable for cycling. Depending on their place of residence (in the suburbs or near downtown), the inhabitants of urban spaces are not equal: they do not all travel the same distances to get to their workplaces or to do their shopping, they do not all have access to the same cycling infrastructures, and do not all face similar road traffic or have to face the same feelings of insecurity when traveling. This reflection also applies to short trips on foot or by bike, which were strongly encouraged during the Covid-19 lockdowns, but whose benefits depended on the characteristics of the neighborhood: in certain neighborhoods with fewer resources favorable to health, these short trips could act as a source of stress and actually have negative health impacts. Promoting the practice of cycling or walking without taking into account the diversity of physical environments as well as the socio-economic contexts of individuals can lead to various forms of exclusion.

Negative effects may also emerge from the increased responsibility that policies promoting physical activity and active mobility place on certain segments of the population. In this sense, we can emphasize that parents and guardians constitute one of the populations particularly targeted by the promotion of physical activity among young people, because they are held responsible for the activities of their children. For example, the Canada 2020 report card emphasized the role of the family in promoting the physical activity of young people (ParticipAction 2020). This report card describes how the family (especially the parents) are a strong source of influence on the active or sedentary behaviors of children (ParticipAction 2020). These recommendations encourage parents to be more active themselves, above all, because their behaviors serve as a model for their children. However, a blind spot appears in the responsibilization of parents: the recommendations do not acknowledge the fact that not all parents or guardians are able to be active in the same way for various reasons and that the impossibility of being an active role model may have a guilt-inducing effect on parents and guardians. Furthermore, when parents or guardians fail to motivate their families or children who like to play alone, sedentarily, or who do not like sports to change their behaviors, this may be experienced by parents or guardians as a failure, or even cause anxiety or feelings of guilt if they interpret this as endangering their family's health (Fullagar 2008). Targeting parents and guardians and prescribing responsibilities for their children's physical activity may have unintended or negative effects.

Finally, it is important to identify the population whose voice or perspective is not heard, even though they constitute the "core target". For instance, there is little consideration given to the voice – or perspective – of children themselves when the physical activity recommendations targeting them are developed and implemented. To make recommendations and interventions more relevant to children and young people, the perspectives and experiences of children from diverse backgrounds should be included (Alexander and Shareck 2021; Gill 2021). In response to this omission, which is becoming more and more obvious, the latest French report card (2020) suggested "conducting a national assessment campaign with parents and youth in order to better appraise, estimate and understand (quantitative and qualitative approach) the importance of outdoor spaces and the urban environment on the physical activity of children and adolescents" (ONAPS 2021, p. 48).

## 6.5. Discussion

This chapter has described public health actions and recommendations concerning physical activity in Canada and France and tried to make the assumptions underlying them more explicit, in order to understand the possible unexpected effects of public health recommendations (Bacchi 2009). As previously mentioned, the "question-posing approach" proposed by Bacchi does not seek to reject recommendations, but rather to highlight certain assumptions and uncover their unintended effects. This approach is particularly important since public health (and its related fields) involves powerful governmental institutions whose values and assumptions acquire widely recognized and accepted legitimacy.

As such, prioritizing certain forms of "healthy" active mobility is not contested in the field of public health. For example, public health discourses mainly value populations (children and their families) who engage in sports or physical activity, who travel on foot or by bicycle. The omnipresence of these discourses on physical activity illustrates the predominance of a biomedical perspective around the population's health and well-being. However, the consequences of this dominant vision should not be neglected. For example, a child whose size deviates from the average size of children their age, or who does not play sports is often perceived as having poor health, and as being at risk of other illnesses, and in need of intervention. Even though these discourses can encourage the physical activity of the majority of the population, they can also lead to the marginalization of certain individuals (children, adults, etc.) who do not fit into the established norms, excluding those who simply do not or cannot engage in recommended forms of physical activity.

This reflection took on particular importance in the context of the Covid-19 pandemic. We may wonder how physical activity and active mobility evolved during the pandemic, and in particular during lockdown periods. Not surprisingly, several studies found a decline in physical activity and an increase in sedentary behavior with the onset of the pandemic (Steckel et al. 2021). How can daily mobility be promoted while preventing recommendations from giving rise to unexpected effects?

As with any health promotion intervention, but especially during the time of Covid-19, we should explicitly recognize that the assumptions underlying interventions have unintended effects, especially because the recommendations to be (and to stay) active during lockdown periods will not be adopted as easily by those who have lesser means to do so. For example, the multiple recommendations to "stay active at home" issued during lockdown were based on the same values and assumptions about physical activity and health as before the Covid-19 pandemic. During lockdown, however, these recommendations were more easily followed by families living in larger houses or those with gardens, or by those with parks, green spaces or playgrounds near their homes (Alexander and Shareck 2021). While the importance of environmental constraints has already been mentioned, these can weigh more heavily during periods when restrictions are imposed on traveling (e.g. travel limited to 1 km around the home during lockdown periods in France): populations are all the more dependent on their immediate environment, which can exacerbate inequalities between families who do or do not have a garden, park, playground or wooded area near their home (Botton 2020) – see Chapter 3.

By offering a critical analysis of the actions and policies promoting physical activity and active mobility, this chapter did not intend to call into question the value of implementing these actions and policies, which are often essential. The goal was rather to discuss the assumptions and implicit values underlying these messages in order to bring awareness of their possible unintended effects on the population. These considerations may help put in place alternative policies that prevent possible negative effects and lead to more inclusive interventions (Alexander et al. 2020).

## 6.6. References

Active Healthy Kids Canada (2005). Dropping the ball/Échapper la balle. Canada's report card on physical activity for children and youth. Report, Active Healthy Kids, Ottawa.

Active Healthy Kids Global Alliance (2020). Active Healthy Kids Global Alliance – Our history [Online]. Available at: https://www.activehealthykids.org/about/#our-history [Accessed 10 May 2020].

Adams, M.L. (2019). Step-counting in the "health-society": Phenomenological reflections on walking in the era of the Fitbit. *Soc. Theory Health*, 17, 109–124. doi: 10.1057/s41285-018-0071-8.

Alexander, S.A. and Shareck, M. (2021). Widening the gap? Unintended consequences of health promotion measures for young people during COVID-19 lockdown. *Health Promotion International.* doi: 10.1093/heapro/daab015.

Alexander, S.A., Frohlich, K.L., Fusco, C. (2014a). Active play may be lots of fun, but it's certainly not frivolous: The emergence of active play as a health practice in Canadian public health. *Sociology of Health & Illness*, 36, 1188–1204. doi: 10.1111/1467-9566.12158.

Alexander, S.A., Frohlich, K.L., Fusco, C. (2014b). Problematizing "Play-for-Health" discourses through children's photo-elicited narratives. *Qualitative Health Research*, 24, 1329–1341. doi: 10.1177/1049732314546753.

Alexander, S.A., Frohlich, K., Fusco, C. (2019). *Play, Physical Activity and Public Health: The Reframing of Children's Leisure Lives.* Routledge/Taylor & Francis Group, London.

Alexander, S.A., Jones, C.M., Tremblay, M.-C., Beaudet, N., Rod, M.H., Wright, M.T. (2020). Reflexivity in health promotion: A typology for training. *Health Promotion Practice.* doi: 10.1177/1524839920912407.

Aubert, S., Barnes, J.D., Forse, M.L., Turner, E., González, S.A., Kalinowski, J., Katzmarzyk, P.T., Lee, E-Y., Ocansey, R., Reilly, J.J. et al. (2019). The international impact of the active healthy kids global alliance physical activity report cards for children and youth. *Journal of Physical Activity and Health*, 16, 679– 697. doi: 10.1123/jpah.2019-0244.

Bacchi, C. (2009). *Analysing Policy: What's the Problem Represented To Be?* Pearson, Frenchs Forest.

Bacchi, C. (2010). Foucault, policy and rule: Challenging the problem-solving paradigm. doi: 10.5278/FREIA.33190049.

Bauman, A., Madill, J., Craig, C.L., Salmon, A. (2004). This mouse roared, but did it get the cheese? *Canadian Journal of Public Health*, 95, S15–S21. doi: 10.1007/BF03403998.

Bletsas, A. and Beasley, C. (eds) (2012). *Engaging with Carol Bacchi: Strategic Interventions and Exchanges.* University of Adelaide Press, Adelaide.

Botton, H. (2020). Accès aux espaces verts : des inégalités révélées par la Covid-19 [Online]. Available at: https://theconversation.com/acces-aux-espaces-verts-des-inegalites-revelees-par-la-covid-19-150864.

Cambon, M., L'Horset, P., Ireps Occitanie (2021). *Promouvoir l'activité physique dans les territoires.* Collection Fnes D-CoDé Santé, Saint-Denis.

Canadian Society for Exercise Physiology (2011). Canadian physical activity guidelines – Key messages. Canadian Society for Exercise Physiology, Ottawa.

Canadian Society for Exercise Physiology (2020). Canadian physical activity guidelines. Canadian Society for Exercise Physiology, Ottawa.

Cavill, N., Kahlmeier, S., Racioppi, F. (2006). Physical activity and health in Europe evidence for action. Report, World Health Organization, Regional Office for Europe, Copenhagen.

Centers for Disease Control and Prevention (1996). Physical activity and health: A report of the surgeon general. Report, Centers for Disease Control and Prevention, Washington.

Edwards, P. (2004). No country mouse: Thirty years of effective marketing and health communications. *Canadian Journal of Public Health*, 95, S6–S13.

Egom, E.E., Pharithi, R.B., Shiwani, H.A., Khan, B., Kruzliak, P., El-Hiani, Y., Maher, V. (2018). Time to redefine body mass index categories in chronic diseases? Spotlight on obesity paradox. *International Journal of Food Sciences and Nutrition*, 69(5), 513–523. doi: 10.1080/09637486.2017.1389859.

Etkin, J. (2016). The hidden cost of personal quantification. *Journal of Consumer Research*, 42, 967–984. doi: 10.1093/jcr/ucv095.

Favier-Ambrosini, B. (2016). Socio-histoire du lien entre activité physique et santé de 1960 à 1980. *Santé Publique*, S1, 13. doi: 10.3917/spub.160.0013.

Flegal, K.M. (2005). Excess deaths associated with underweight, overweight, and obesity. *JAMA*, 293, 1861. doi: 10.1001/jama.293.15.1861

Flegal, K.M., Graubard, B.I., Williamson, D.F., Gail, M.H. (2007). Cause-specific excess deaths associated with underweight, overweight, and obesity. *JAMA*, 298(17), 2028. doi: 10.1001/jama.298.17.2028.

Foucault, M. (1997). *La volonté de savoir : histoire de la sexualité.* Gallimard, Paris.

French Ministry of Ecological Transition (2019). Le plan vélo et mobilités actives. Report, Government of the French Republic, Paris.

French Ministry of Solidarity and Health (2019). Programme national Nutrution santé 2019–2023. Report, Government of the French Republic, Paris.

Fullagar, S. (2008). Governing healthy family lifestyles through discourses of risk and responsibility. In *Biopolitics and the Obesity Epidemic: Governing Bodies*, Wright, J. and Harwood, V. (eds). Routledge, London.

Gard, M. and Wright, J. (2001). Managing uncertainty: Obesity discourses and physical education in a risk society. *Studies in Philosophy and Education*, 20, 535–549. doi: 10.1023/A:1012238617836.

Gill, T. (2021). *Urban Playground: How Child-Friendly Planning and Design can Save Cities*. RIBA Publishing, London.

Gutin, I. (2018). In BMI we trust: Reframing the body mass index as a measure of health. *Social Theory & Health*, 16(3), 256–271. doi: 10.1057/s41285-017-0055-0.

Haut Conseil de la Santé Publique (2018). Prévention et promotion de la santé. Une responsabilité collective. *La Revue ADSP*, 103, 64.

Humphreys, S. (2010). The unethical use of BMI in contemporary general practice. *British Journal of General Practice*, 60, 696–697. doi: 10.3399/bjgp10X515548.

Institut national de la santé et de la recherche médicale (Inserm) (2008). Activité physique : contextes et effets sur la santé. Report, Les éditions Inserm, Paris.

LeBesco, K. (2011). Neoliberalism, public health, and the moral perils of fatness. *Critical Public Health*, 21, 153–164. doi: 10.1080/09581596.2010.529422.

Lemonnier, F., Van Hoye, A., Furrer, P., Bunde-Birouste, A.W., Rostan, F. (2020). Promouvoir la santé par l'activité sportive et physique. *La santé en action*, 454.

McCartney, M. and Bauld, L. (2019). The great obesity debate: Divided we fall. *The Lancet Gastroenterology & Hepatology*, 4, 655. doi: 10.1016/S2468-1253 (19)30229-8.

Moffat, T. (2010). The "childhood obesity epidemic". *Medical Anthropology Quarterly*, 24, 1–21. doi: 10.1111/j.1548-1387.2010.01082.x.

Noël Racine, A., Van Hoye, A., Baron, A., Lecomte, F., Garbarino, J.-M., Massiera, B., Honta, M., Vuillemin, A. (2021). Development of a local health-enhancing physical activity policy analysis tool in France: CAPLA-Santé. *Health Promotion Practice*, 22, 540–548. doi: 10.1177/1524839920916462.

ONAPS (2016). Report Card. Activité physique et sédentarité de l'enfant et adolescent : premier état des lieux en France [Online]. Available at: https://onaps.fr/report-card-sur-lactivite-physique-et-la-sedentarite-de-lenfant-et-adolescent/.

ONAPS (2020). ONAPS Actualités [Online]. Available at: http://www.onaps.fr/.

ONAPS (2021). Activité physique et sédentarité de l'enfant et de l'adolescent : nouvel état des lieux en France [Online]. Available at: https://onaps.fr/wp-content/uploads/2022/10/RC_2022-web-vflight.pdf.

ParticipACTION (2020). Le rôle de la famille dans l'activité physique, les comportements sédentaires et le sommeil des enfants et des jeunes. Bulletin de l'activité physique chez les enfants et les jeunes de ParticipACTION. Report, ParticipACTION, Ottawa.

Praznoczy, C., Lambert, C., Pascal, C. (2017). État des lieux de l'activité physique et de la sédentarité en France. Report, French National Observatory for Physical Activity and Sedentary Behaviors, Clermont-Ferrand.

Prévot-Ledrich, J., Van Hoye, A., Lombrail, P., Lecomte, F., Vuillemin, A. (2016). Panorama des politiques publiques françaises de promotion de l'activité physique bénéfique pour la santé. *Santé Publique*, S1, 25–31. doi: 10.3917/spub.160.0025.

Rostan, F., Simon, C., Ulmer, Z. (2011). Promouvoir l'activité physique des jeunes. Élaborer et développer un projet de type Icaps. Institut national de prévention et d'éducation pour la santé, Saint-Denis.

Sharratt, M.T. and Hearst, W.E. (2007). Canada's physical activity guides: Background, process, and development. *Applied Physiology, Nutrition, and Metabolism*, 32, S9–S15. doi: 10.1139/H07-124.

Stockwell, S., Trott, M., Tully, M., Shin, J., Barnett, Y., Butler, L., McDermott, D., Schuch, F., Smith, L. (2021). Changes in physical activity and sedentary behaviours from before to during the COVID-19 pandemic lockdown: A systematic review. *BMJ Open Sport & Exercise Medicine*, 7, e000960. doi: 10.1136/bmjsem-2020-000960.

Thibault, H., Duché, P., Meyer, M., Pérès, G., Association pour la prévention et la prise en charge de l'obésité en pédiatrie (APOP) (2008). Activité physique et obésité de l'enfant. Bases pour une prescription adaptée. Report, Programme Nationale Nutrition Santé, Besançon.

Tremblay, M.S., LeBlanc, A.G., Carson, V., Choquette, L., Connor Gorber, S., Dillman, C., Duggan, M., Gordon, M.J., Hicks, A., Janssen, I., et al. (2012). Canadian physical activity guidelines for the early years (aged 0–4 years). *Appl. Physiol. Nutr. Metab.*, 37, 345–356. doi: 10.1139/h2012-018.

Tremblay, M.S., Barnes, J.D., Bonne, J.C. (2014). Impact of the Active Healthy Kids Canada report card: A 10-year analysis. *Journal of Physical Activity and Health*, 11, S3–S20. doi: 10.1123/jpah.2014-0167.

United Nations Children's Fund (2012). The state of the world's children 2012: Children in an urban world. Report, UNICEF, New York.

Veronese, N., Cereda, E., Solmi, M., Fowler, S.A., Manzato, E., Maggi, S., Manu, P., Abe, E., Hayashi, K., Allard, J.P. et al. (2015). Inverse relationship between body mass index and mortality in older nursing home residents: A meta-analysis of 19,538 elderly subjects: BMI and mortality in nursing home. *Obesity Reviews*, 16(11), 1001–1015. doi: 10.1111/obr.12309.

Vuillemin, A. (2018). Activité physique – dossiers documentaires de la Société française de santé publique. Créer des conditions favorables à l'activité physique : connaissances, stratégies et interventions [Online]. Available at: https://www.sfsp.fr/content-page/item/3096-activite-physique-3096 [Accessed 9 October 2020].

WHO French Healthy Cities Network (2013). *Mobilités actives au quotidien : le rôle des collectivités.* Presses de l'EHESP, Rennes.

World Health Organization (2010). Recommandations mondiales sur l'activité physique pour la santé. Report, WHO, Geneva.

World Health Organization (2015). Comité régional de l'Europe. Stratégie sur l'activité physique pour la région européenne de l'OMS 2016-2025. Report, WHO Europe, Copenhagen.

World Health Organization (2016). Report of the commission on ending childhood obesity. WHO, Geneva.

World Health Organization (2018). More active people for a healthier world: Global action plan on physical activity 2018–2030. WHO, Geneva.

World Health Organization (2020). Lignes directrices de l'OMS sur l'activité physique et la sédentarité : en un coup d'œil. Report, WHO, Geneva.

# 7

# Rationalization of the Healthcare Provision and Mobility

**Véronique LUCAS-GABRIELLI**[1] **and Catherine MANGENEY**[2,3]

[1] *Irdes, Paris, France*

[2] *ORS Île-de-France, Paris, France*

[3] *Géographie-cités, Université Paris Cité, France*

## 7.1. Introduction

After World War II, the development of health systems with a universal vocation in Europe initially took place in a context of reconstruction and a growing economy. This enabled social progress and concomitantly fueled economic growth. In France, as in other developed countries, many hospitals were created and the number of doctors increased. This led to an increase in the weight of the health sector on the economy (Palier 2017).

Several major changes led all developed countries to change the organization of their healthcare system. In the early 1970s, in a context of economic crisis, controlling the expansion of health systems became crucial to harness the budgets associated with them. System efficiency was sought, particularly as an unequal distribution of sanitary equipment and services had been identified (Barer and Stoddart 1992; Kervasdoué and Picheral 2004; Bourgueil et al. 2006; Bailoni 2011).

*Everyday Mobility and Health*,
coordinated by Julie VALLÉE. 

Systems for regulating the healthcare provision were placed in all developed countries. Whatever form this regulation takes in correlation with the specificity of the different national healthcare systems, the question arises as to the development of a system of spatialized standards to establish:

– the indicators for the territorial monitoring of the adequacy between the population's healthcare needs and health resources;

– the thresholds below which this adequacy is considered not to have been achieved and beyond which the situation may be deemed acceptable;

– the territorial divisions to target public action on so-called priority territories.

As regards healthcare provision planning – the act of setting goals for the harmonious distribution of equipment and services required for the well-being of populations and the efficiency of these activities (Merlin and Choay 2010) – regulatory policies are developed, in the sense of all the processes making it possible to preserve the essential balance of an organized system, formed by interdependent and interacting elements and permanently subject to external disturbances (Chevalier 2004). These regulatory policies feed the rationalization of healthcare based on territorial divisions deemed to be the best suited to support the regulatory goal.

This chapter specifically focuses on healthcare rationalization policies: it will present the way in which these rationalization policies (which are part of a global movement of public policy territorialization) have been constructed and have evolved over time. It will also shed light on the development of these technologies and evaluate to what extent they integrate the questions of daily mobility of populations.

In terms of healthcare planning, the chapter will first introduce the approaches that measure spatial accessibility to healthcare in terms of the distance between the population and the healthcare provision (section 7.2). Then, it will detail the way in which population mobility is taken into consideration (or not) by spatial accessibility to healthcare and in the delimitation of territories when planning the healthcare provision. We will begin with an appraisal of the traditional density (section 7.3) and distance (section 7.4) indicators. While the former do not take mobility into account, the latter only consider it in terms of distance. We will then discuss the methodologies for delimiting health planning territories based on journey flows (section 7.5) and the most recent methods for measuring spatial accessibility to healthcare by means of an encompassing approach to mobility, combining availability and distance via gravity models on the influence of provision (section 7.6). Before concluding, we will present the current organizational transformations of the healthcare system which seem to conceal (at least partly) the concept of mobility in healthcare provision planning policies, while favoring coordination among actors (section 7.7).

## 7.2. Spatial accessibility at the heart of healthcare rationalization policies

Healthcare rationalization policies aim to improve the organization of the healthcare system within an increasingly constrained budgetary framework for most countries. They are based on an estimate of the adequacy between the level of care offered and the care needs of populations. They are also based on the measurement of accessibility to resources, including spatial[1] accessibility, which has been the subject of many studies in the fields of transport, urban planning, food, employment and healthcare (Peng 1997; Geurs and Van Wee 2004; Charreire et al. 2010; Cheng and Bertolini 2013).

The notion of spatial accessibility covers the greater or lesser ease with which places, people or activities can be reached (Bavoux and Chapelon 2015). In practice, spatial accessibility measures focus on one or more components of accessibility, depending on perspective. Four types of approach result from this (Geurs and Van Wee 2004):

– the first type of approach measures the efficiency of transport networks; it relies on indicators such as traffic congestion or average travel speed, for example;

– the second type of approach concerns measures focusing on places that characterize accessibility in terms of the physical distance between the location of services and the places of origin (key locations of daily life such as place of residence or workplace, for example). These measurements provide essential information in terms of territorial allocation when planning

1. Spatial accessibility is only one of the dimensions of accessibility, alongside temporal, financial, cultural and social accessibility. Temporal accessibility mainly refers to policies for organizing the permanence of care, whereas financial accessibility is considered through the use of tools such as complementary universal health insurance (CMU, *Complémentaire maladie universelle*), the regulation of medical expenses, care and drug reimbursements, etc.

the provision (Apparicio et al. 2008) and can be implemented operationally by working with existing databases and algorithms;

– the third approach, based on the concept of time-geography (Hägerstrand 1970), expresses accessibility as the spatio-temporal constraints of individuals (Chardonnel 2007; Kwan 2004; Ellegård and Svedin 2012);

– in the last type of approach, accessibility is understood on the basis of the benefit individuals derive from the access to services by calculating the probability of an individual making a particular choice based on the relative utility they attribute to that choice, compared to all other possible choices.

If, as Fol and Gallez (2013) point out, an ideal measure of accessibility should take into account these four approaches, accessibility is nonetheless a difficult concept to translate into operational indicators (Handy and Niemeier 1997). In terms of healthcare resource planning, the measurement of disparities in accessibility between territories is often basic or incomplete: it essentially replicates measurement focusing on places. Moreover, the link between the analytical scale of territorial disparities and the operational scale of planning is only rarely called into question (see Conclusion). The notion of spatial accessibility is key in the field of healthcare planning, particularly with a view to ensuring greater equity between citizens in their potential to reach sanitary facilities and services. Here, the notion is called upon bearing in mind John Rawls'[2] goal of social and spatial justice. Although it does not encompass Amartya Sen's notion of capability (in its normative form, directly translatable in terms of political goals), it nonetheless makes it possible to understand socio-spatial inequalities as opportunities and potentialities (Fol and Gallez 2013). However, for a certain spatial context, it would still be necessary to develop empirical and qualitative studies on the way in which people may or may not appropriate the potential for accessibility available to them (Fol and Gallez 2013).

From a basic and operational point of view, different methodologies for measuring place-based healthcare accessibility can be identified. The first (traditionally used) one associates the healthcare provision of a geographical entity with its resident population (density indicators) or measures the

2. The work on social justice developed by Rawls advocates a fair distribution of primary goods (guaranteeing access to the poorest). Amartya Sen, for his part, offers a broader vision and encourages us to consider not only the possibilities offered to individuals, but also the variation in their capabilities to mobilize them.

remoteness to the provision for an individual or a population (distance indicators) (Luo and Wang 2003; Ricketts 2010). Gravity models on the influence of provision have then been developed, combining distance and availability (Talen and Anselin 1998; Apparicio et al. 2008; McGrail and Humphreys 2009c). Indeed, the presence of a health service is not enough to ensure spatial accessibility to healthcare. This service must be made available, which means that it needs to have sufficient appointment slots to meet the population's needs. It should be noted that this is only a matter of potential spatial accessibility, which does not include the other possible obstacles to accessibility (temporal, financial, social or cultural).

All of these spatial accessibility measurement indicators used for implementing the planning, regulation and rationalization policies of sanitary equipment and services rely on the concept of mobility in a differentiated way.

## 7.3. Density indicators: mobility left aside

The medical density indicator is the ratio between the number of practitioners and the population. Stricto sensu, it expresses a rate rather than a density (which denotes the relationship between a number of individuals or objects and a surface). The term "physician-to-population ratio" used by English-speaking countries is, in this way, the more appropriate term rather than the commonly used expression "medical density" (Picheral 2001). This medical density indicator is widely used. It has the advantage of being easily calculable and intuitive for professionals and decision-makers, while being based on readily available data. Healthcare provision ratios (densities) are traditionally used in the international comparison of health systems to highlight the differences in allocations between countries or between types of space within each country (urban vs. rural setting) (OECD 2016; European Observatory on Health Systems and Policies 2020). In the same way, it is frequently used in national analyses to measure staffing disparities at different scales and to set equipment and professional standard rates within the framework of planning or regulation exercises conducted by the national or local authorities. It has also been used for delimiting territories or to encourage health professionals to settle in a specific place.

In France, for example, between the 1970s and the 1990s, the regulation of hospital provision was based on respect of ratios: bed provision ranges per medical discipline or equipment defined at the national level and applied at the local level for each health sector. In Belgium, the demarcation of priority areas facing a shortage of general practitioners is based on a medical density threshold: a region is considered to have a shortage if the number of general practitioners for every 100,000 inhabitants is lower than 90 (Missinne and Luyten 2018).

Depending on the healthcare provision considered, its level of specialization and the equipment cost, the healthcare[3] network gradation principle implies that certain services must be accessible nearby (general practitioners in particular) while others (highly specialized ones) can be located remotely (heart transplant service, for example). Again, the scale of analysis used must be more or less detailed depending on the healthcare provision considered: interregional, regional or intermediate level for hospital equipment, smaller administrative entities for primary care (*Kreis* in Germany; the *bassin de vie* and the pseudo-canton in France).

In all cases in which density indicators are involved, the mobility of populations is not considered within the geographical entity of analysis, at both the largest and the finest scales. In this respect, not only is mobility between units of analysis not considered, but mobility within each unit of analysis is viewed as negligible.

In other words, density primarily refers to the availability of the healthcare provision in a given territory. This implicitly assumes that the service or professional located on the other side of the zone boundary will be unreachable. It ignores population movements (even though they are frequent) across administrative boundaries, especially for density measured in small areas (Salze et al. 2011).

Second, density-type indicators consider that within the same entity of analysis, the entire care supply is accessible to the inhabitants, including when the entity of analysis is as vast as a region. As a result, another limitation of this type of indicator concerns its high sensitivity to the size and configuration of the chosen spatial unit (Modified Areal Unit Problem, MAUP effect) described in many works (Openshaw 1984; Mathian and Sanders 2006; Apparicio et al. 2008). This spatial unit is rarely defined in

3. For example, this principle was explicitly defined for the first time in France in Circular No. 101 of March 5, 2004, which proposed a gradation of care into five levels, each corresponding to different types of care and a particular geographic scale: levels of proximity, intermediatry, recourse catchment area, regional and interregional levels.

close relation to mobility and is factually constrained by data availability (often provided at various administrative levels, rather than at observation levels better suited to this type of exercise).

Finally, density indicators do not take into account the specific and differentiated needs of populations, which leads health authorities to combine them with other socio-demographic indicators.

For example, while simple healthcare provision ratios per capita were used in the United States (Ricketts et al. 2007) in the 1970s to identify areas with a shortage of primary healthcare (the threshold initially adopted being full-time medical equivalent for every 4,000 inhabitants), these were quickly combined with other socio-demographic indicators such as infant mortality rate, percentage of 65+ patients and the population share living below the poverty line. Following the same goal of taking into account the differentiated needs of populations, the delimitation of sectors lacking in general practitioners followed an identical course in France in the 2000s. As for Germany, medical provision planning is based on an indicator conveying the number of doctors required to meet the population's needs. This threshold is calculated on the basis of several criteria (demography, existing offer, morbidity, distances). A district is closed to all settlements if the number of physicians practicing there exceeds the defined need by over 10%. On the contrary, settlements are encouraged for practitioners in areas with fewer resources (Hassenteufel et al. 2020).

The need to combine medical densities with other indicators reflecting the heterogeneity of populations and their needs reflects the operational limits of density indicators. However, the use of composite indicators of this type dilutes the nature of the statistical instrument, which no longer makes it possible to distinguish (Ricketts et al. 2007) between problems in the distribution of healthcare provision and social inequalities in health. In the United States (Ricketts et al. 2007) as well as in France (Barlet et al. 2012), research has sought to improve the quantification of the numerator (healthcare provision volume) and the denominator (care needs) by analyzing the provision actually available (or accessible), by weighing the population by sex, age and/or social characteristics. Still, the provision/need ratios neglect the mobility factors that make it possible to look at the provision against needs.

## 7.4. The distance indicators: the concept of accessibility is introduced by traveling

Distances make it possible to locate populations who live far from healthcare services. Therefore, distance is a fundamental dimension of accessibility. The development of Geographic Information Systems (GIS), which multiply the possibilities offered in terms of calculations, has improved their measurement from Euclidean distances (length of a line segment between two points) to reticular distances (following the network route) or, more recently, time-distances. Time-distances are distances expressed in minutes rather than kilometers (time required to get from point A to point B, taking into account the road network or transport infrastructure and depending on a specific mode of transport, most often the private car).

In Sweden, for example, "when economically and geographically possible", the government recommends primary care centers to be "easily reachable", which, in calculation models, is expressed by the idea that no inhabitant should travel over 30 km by road to reach the nearest center (provided that centers can also achieve the minimum level of patient attendance) (Aschan-Leygonia 2017).

Distances are used as a performance indicator for the allocation of resources in the territory. Distance control and reduction constitute a permanent concern in terms of healthcare provision planning. Distance reduction also has to be compatible with the proximity/safety/quality triptych as well as with budgetary equilibrium. In particular, this arbitration arises for certain services such as primary care provision, maternity wards, digestive surgery or even orthopedics, not to mention ophthalmology or gynecology, which are hospital disciplines with high demand both in terms of urgent and scheduled care.

Hospital location models (Gould and Leinbach 1966; Morrill and Earickson 1969; Thouez 1987) have sought to minimize the distances to be traveled for a maximum number of patients in a given territory. Nevertheless, the contribution of this type of analysis, which generally simplifies the methodological hypotheses formulated, has often been called into question (Coldefy and Lefebvre 2019; Meade and Earickson 2000). Typically, patient behavior is often considered to be homogeneous, with the assumption that patients will use the closest service to their home and that demand for care and its provision, can be calculated without consideration of their respective characteristics (Rosenberg 1988). However, for healthcare provision, as for many other services, the use of the nearest service is not the norm. For general practitioners alone, the work of Gravelle (1996) showed that only one-third of the patients were appointed to the general practitioner closest to them. Other studies have confirmed that patients do not attend the closest, but one of the closest services (Hays et al. 1990; Forzy et al. 2021). The reasons are previous contacts with the doctor, recommendations from other general practitioners, or cultural, religious or ethnic factors. For other types of care, such as hospital care, proximity is only the third reason for choice, after reputation and medical advice (Lacoste and Spinosi 2002). Furthermore, distance is plural in the sense of the possible metrics (Lévy and Lussault 2013) and the various forms (physical, social, perceived) used for expressing it.

The plural approach to distance refers to the variations observed in the trips made by individuals. Travel is conditioned by the spatial distribution of the resources to be reached (physical distance), the performance of the transport infrastructure and the "mobility potential or capital" of individuals – their "motility" (Kaufmann 2001). The individuals' characteristics such as income level, age, gender, social origin, physical or cognitive skills (Guagliardo 2004) influence "the capacity [of individuals] to use certain modes of transport or services, their degree of discrimination in relation to certain activities or individual constraints systems" (Fol and Gallez 2013), all of which can lead to social distance from resources. In addition, these individual characteristics as well as daily life habits influence the way in which each individual evaluates the distance to resources, that is, the perceived distance (Charron and Shearmur 2005): healthcare facilities located close to different daily life places seem more accessible and more reachable than others (Cromley and Shannon 1986). Insofar as these physical, social and perceived distances arise from relationships between individuals and healthcare structures located in space, the distance metrics used for measuring accessibility should take into account the diversity of populations and territories.

## 7.5. The use of travel flows to define planning territories

Journeys towards healthcare services have long been studied in order to describe the use of services and to measure the impact of accessibility on effective access to care (Joseph and Phillips 1984; Hunter et al. 1986;

Carr-Hill et al. 1997; Lucas-Gabrielli et al. 2016). They have also been used for defining support territories for the organization of care activities (Vigneron and Brau 1996).

Mobility is characterized through the prism of patients' traveling practices towards health professionals and care structures, which can all be located, spatialized and mapped (Bonerandi 2004). These flows were used for highlighting if comparable use behavior of groups of individuals could be identified according to a spatial criterion. On the basis of these flows, some researchers proposed to define "service areas" or "health catchment areas"[4] (Vigneron and Corvez 1999; Macé 2002). Defined as a spatial container, these "catchment areas" served as support for healthcare planning (in particular, in the regional schemes for the organization of care regarding hospital planning in France) or sometimes for the delimitation of compulsory healthcare recourse areas (e.g. some managed care plans in the United States).

The use of healthcare flows as support for health planning does however raises a certain number of objections. A first limitation concerns the fact that indicators based on healthcare consumption data alone confirm the shortcomings and do not take non-use into account (Rican and Vaillant 2009). A second limitation relates to the fact of considering the population's choices to be rational, whereas attraction is a complex phenomenon. It depends on many parameters such as the distance and provision availability, as well as its price, quality or reputation (Cromley and McLafferty 2002). Finally, another limitation concerns the difficulty of accounting for the complexity of flows in the face of a wide variety of patient behaviors. Most often, only the main flows are used for building catchment areas or areas of attractiveness, which does not reflect the dispersion of consumption flows. On the contrary, when all the flows are considered, the geography they draw is complex and interwoven, especially in dense and multi-polarized areas. In this type of area, daily mobility, like less frequent mobility (to healthcare in particular), is organized according to complex and highly intertwined individual strategies (Bouleau and Mangeney 2015) (Figure 7.1).

4. Comparatively, the gravity models of Reilly (1963) and Huff (1964) have often been used for defining theoretical hospital areas of attraction that overlook the actual behavior of the population in terms of traveling and the recourse to services. These behaviors may differ from the "logical" recourse that these methods provide for various reasons (reputation of establishments, patient referral, etc.).

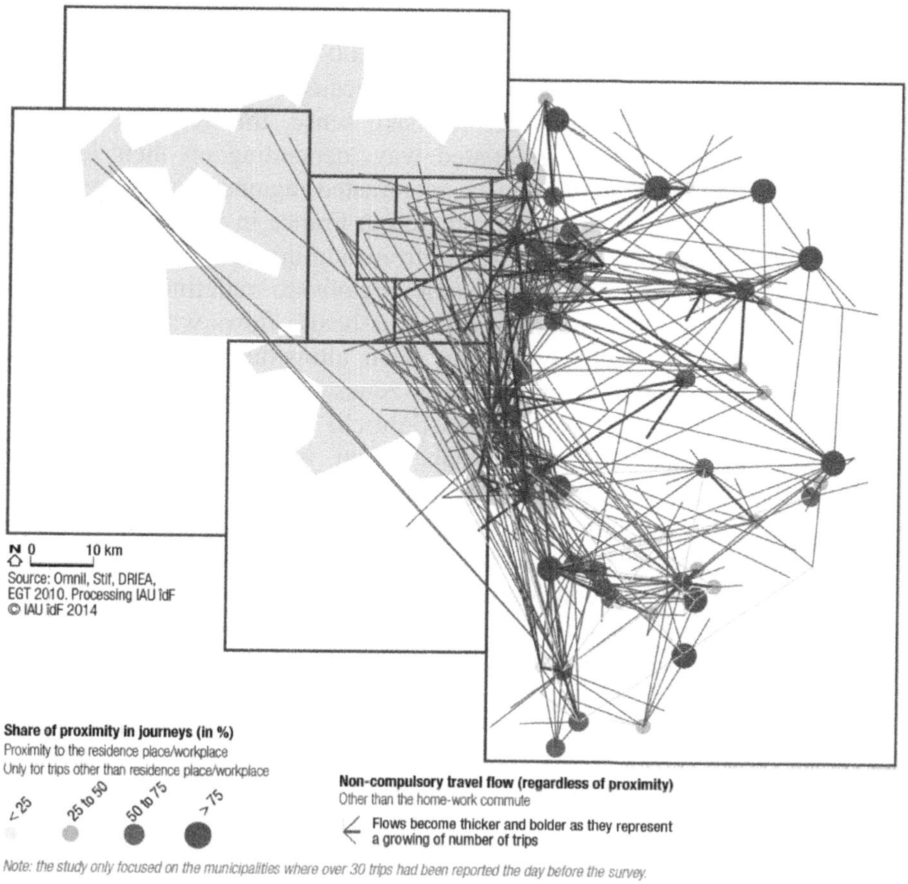


**Figure 7.1.** *Schematic geography of non-compulsory travel in an Île-de-France department (source: Bouleau and Mangeney 2015). For a color version of this figure, see www.iste.co.uk/vallee/everyday.zip*

COMMENT ON FIGURE 7.1.– *Scope: journeys of residents from Seine-et-Marne surveyed in the 2010 Global Transport Survey – journeys made the day before the day of the survey – every trip considered, except the "compulsory" ones (returns home or commuting to work or to the study place). The brown rectangles schematically represent the eight departments of Île-de-France.*

To go beyond approaches that focus only on the sanitary flows, home–work commuting or flows to other facilities and services are sometimes taken into account to define "living" territories, close to daily mobility or habitual mobility spaces (Julien 2007) and considered relevant territories for the organization of healthcare because they are legitimized by the inhabitants' practices. In order to make sense, this requires thinking about health territories in a graduated way, depending on their level of specialization, so that they can be contrasted against territories of a "comparable size". This exercise, promoted in France in the early 2000s by national authorities, to free themselves from administrative territories and acknowledge "local realities", led some regions to redefine their health planning territories. They sought to articulate health flows with other living territories or to free themselves from them altogether by using a more generalist division, such as employment zones or *bassins de vie* ("living catchment areas") (Coldefy and Lucas-Gabrielli 2010). This was the case, for example, for the Nord-Pas-de-Calais region, which chose to define the healthcare provision[5] quantified goals in a differentiated way depending on hospital disciplines, whether at the departmental level, at the level of the living catchment area or at the level of the proximity area (grouping several municipalities). Without considering one to prevail over the others, the comparison of divisions was useful for raising awareness on "the art of division" (Brunet 1997), insofar as the unique and perfectly rational network does not exist.

## 7.6. Floating sector methods: greater integration of mobility

Traditional density and nearest distance indicators have been gradually supplemented by the journeys made by the population. However, public policies for rationalizing and planning the healthcare provision based on these methodologies were quickly denounced on the grounds that they are based on the journeys actually made while confirming shortcomings and overlooking unmet needs. In the 2000s, methodologies were developed to measure accessibility levels to care by two-step floating catchment area (2SFCA) algorithms (Radke and Mu 2000; Luo and Wang 2003; Wang and Luo 2005; Tao et al. 2018). These algorithms are derived from gravity models and close to the "distributed density" model (Mizrahi and Mizrahi 2010). Even though they require some adjustment, the indicators calculated

5. Healthcare quantified goals characterize the distribution of the healthcare provision in each health territory per care activity. Goals are defined according to multi-annual contracts and the means of each health establishment to meet the goals of the territory's medical project in accordance with the resources negotiated with the regional health agency.

in that way have elicited growing interest from the international geographical literature (Allan 2014; Neutens 2015). This methodology has established itself in the French institutional landscape since 2017, when it served as the basis for the definition of zoning areas lacking in health professionals (general practitioners, nurses, masseurs–physiotherapists, etc.) (Box 7.1).

> Since 2017, the delimitation of regulatory zones targeting territories that lack general practitioners was carried out in two stages: first, the 2SFCA methodology was applied for calculating a Local Potential Accessibility indicator (LPA) for each municipality, which was then averaged by "healthy living territories"[6]. Depending on this indicator, the regions were allocated a maximum population quota who could live in an under-provided area.
>
> Considering this quota, the Regional Health Agencies (ARS, *Agences régionales de santé*) have to select a certain number of territories regarded as lacking general practitioners within their region, ranked according to their level of priority (priority intervention zones, complementary action zone and vigilance zones).
>
> Since 2021, the selection of these territories has been at the discretion of the ARS, whether for the ranking of health living areas based on the LPA indicator or "a different ranking from the one resulting from the LPA, provided that the territory's characteristics justify that choice" (French Decree of October 1, 2021)[7].

**Box 7.1.** *Delimitation of French deficit zones lacking in health professionals*

6. Healthy living territories are made up of a group of municipalities. Their delimitation is primarily based on INSEE's "living catchment areas" (division of the national territory into a network of the smallest groupings of municipalities in which inhabitants have access to the most common equipment and services). As the division into living catchment areas deems urban units indivisible, some living catchment areas may comprise over 50,000 inhabitants. Healthy living territories propose a division of these highly populated catchment areas based on similar criteria as for the definition and attractiveness of service hubs. The LPA indicator calculated at the level of the health living territory is the average (weighted by the population of each municipality) of LPA indicators from the municipalities in this territory.

7. French Decree of October 1, 2021 relating to the methodology applicable to the medical profession for determining the areas provided for in no. 1 of Article L. 1434-4 from the Public Health Code.

Under the assumption that a population's demand for a healthcare practitioner does not solely depend on the distance between population and practitioner, but varies depending on the practitioner's availability and the distance from other practitioners (Wan et al. 2012; Luo 2014), these methodologies seek to combine distance and availability and to measure a "potentially" accessible level of provision. To do this, they rely on two hypotheses. The first one is that any inhabitant can potentially use all of the medical services, including those relatively far away and outside their administrative perimeter, but that the probability of use decreases with distance. The second one states that health professionals divide their activity among all the patients who could potentially use their services. Their availability for everyone therefore decreases in proportion to the volume of their potential patient base.

This type of measurement is calculated in two stages. In the first stage, the medical provision is distributed across the practitioner's patient area (defined by the residential sectors located around the medical provision within a certain distance) in proportion to the number of patients sharing it (the method for calculating the probability of recourse may vary from author to author). In the second stage, for each residential sector, the different portions of the medical provision are summed. The indicator obtained has the advantage of expressing the provision density per inhabitant and can be easily appropriated by public decision-makers.

In the very beginning, 2SFCA-type indicators were calculated with the assumption that accessibility was identical for all inhabitants within the area of recourse, but non-existent beyond. These first indicators were later improved based on time-distances and in order to decrease the probability of recourse, either gradually (Luo and Qi 2009) or continuously (Dai and Wang 2011).

However, different studies have identified an over/under-estimation of healthcare accessibility levels using these methodologies, inspired by 2SFCA methods (Wan et al. 2012; Luo 2014; Jamtsho et al. 2015; Li et al. 2015; Neutens 2015), for two main reasons.

The first obstacle is that these methods take little account of absolute remoteness from care. To better describe the system's overall efficiency, Delamater (2013) has proposed a "Modifiable 2SFCA", introducing a modulation factor for the provision/need relationship and pondering it by absolute and relative distance[8]. The underlying hypothesis is that poorly distributed provision will not be entirely consumed by the population.

The second obstacle is that these methods assign the needs of all the inhabitants in each entity of residence to each medical provision, solely on the basis of distance. In particular, they do not take into account the fact that the healthcare demand will be distributed among all these offers. The three-step indicator (3SFCA) proposed by Luo (2014) takes into account the system's chain effects (Li et al. 2015), which translates into the fact that additional provision at a given place will modify the recourse behavior of the inhabitants residing nearby, potentially freeing up "places" for inhabitants living elsewhere, etc.

According to the literature, another limitation of 2SFCA-inspired indicators lies in the fact that the decrease in the probability of recourse according to distance is assumed to be identical for all populations, regardless of their individual characteristics and the nature of their areas of residence (dense urban, peri-urban or rural).

Nevertheless, McGrail (2012) has pointed out that authors whose field of study focuses on an urbanized metropolis make the hypothesis that the recourse to healthcare decreases with the distance more rapidly than the authors studying healthcare accessibility in rural or remote areas. Regardless of the services considered, the inhabitants of rural areas "in the real world" (Wang 2012) always travel greater distances than the inhabitants of dense areas, within which urban amenities are more concentrated.

The Australian authors McGrail and Humphreys (2009a, 2009b, 2009c, 2014) have integrated hypotheses of decreasing recourse according to various distances depending on the urban morphology of territories (more restricted recourse distances in dense urban zones, wider in the margins of agglomerations and even more distended in the most isolated areas). They combine this with a threshold effect limiting the extent of the areas of

8. The notions of absolute/relative distance developed by Delamater refer to the fact that 2SFCA-type methods proceed from a distribution of the provision across populations, by weighting the provision allocated to the different places of residence following the "relative distance" criterion: the populations closest to the healthcare provision will be considered to be more in line with this offer than the furthest populations. However, 2SFCA-type methods do not draw a distinction between situations in which all the places of residence are located at the same distance from healthcare provision, regardless of whether this distance is short (proximity) or long (remote). This is what Delamater calls "absolute distance".

recourse according to the number of medical opportunities reached: only the 100 closest medical provision proposals are considered likely to be chosen by the individuals.

For their part, for stage 1, Luo and Whippo (2012) increase patient areas until a population threshold is reached. For stage 2, they extend recourse areas until a certain provision volume per inhabitant is reached. On their part, Jamtsho, Corner and Dewan (2015) propose patient and recourse areas to be defined by criteria based on the number of closest physicians rather than using time–distance criteria.

However, if used for rationalizing the healthcare provision, these approaches assume that it is politically acceptable to consider that the inhabitants of rural areas have lower proximity needs than the inhabitants of denser areas in terms of access to healthcare. In countries such as Canada (37.4 million inhabitants over 10 million square kilometers) or Australia (25.2 million inhabitants over 7.7 million square kilometers), where spatial configurations and rural or desert areas are extensive, this approach cannot be avoided. In a country like France (64.6 million inhabitants over 0.6 million square kilometers), where areas are smaller and where the equal treatment of citizens is one of the republican pillars, such a presupposition could be politically dangerous.

All of the *x*SFCA-type indicators are based on a modeling of the potentialities offered by the daily mobility of individuals. Dissociating themselves from effective recourse methods, these indicators relate supply and demand in a global system of potentialities governed by recourse probabilities that both depend on the provision distribution in relation to the demand and the effects of competition or choice between care providers, on the one hand, and care seekers, on the other hand. In a largely identical manner, mobility is reduced to an economic criterion (the rationality of travel depending on quantifiable and objective factors, absolute and/or relative distance here replacing the cost of travel, which is dear to economists).

The development of Geographic Information Systems (GIS), localized databases and modeling of reticular distances (distances calculated on the basis of the road network) and time-distances between the different points of a geographic space has made it possible to refine this understanding of spatial mobility in spatial accessibility to care indicators. Thus, Local Potential Accessibility (LPA), a French version of the 2SFCA used for the delimitation of regulatory zoning of the primary care provision (Barlet et al. 2012; Vergier and Chaput 2017), bases its decrease function not on distance separating supply and demand in kilometers but over the time required for an inhabitant to access the healthcare provision by traveling in a private car under average congestion or traffic flow conditions.

Some authors (Mao and Nekorchuk 2013; Langford et al. 2016) have also proposed refining the methodology for calculating the indicator by combining different modes of transport, and no longer restricting it to the sole use of the private car. Populations and distances are weighted according to modal shares (public transport and private car) observed in transport surveys or according to household motorization rates. However, this methodological advance requires the availability of two distinct distance–time matrices, one for the private car, and another for public transport. The latter is often quite difficult to build in the absence of a competent public transport organizing authority throughout the national territory. On the contrary, these authors have shown that this integration of multiple modes of transport affects results in rural areas to a small extent (because the majority of journeys are made by car), whereas results change significantly in dense areas, where the use of public transport is much more widespread. Research carried out in Île-de-France (Lucas-Gabrielli and Mangeney 2019) seems to indicate that the integration of multi-modality does not upset major balances – even in the dense Île-de-France zone – but rather modifies them in a sensitive manner at the local level.

The work of Lucas-Gabrielli and Mangeney (2019) has also shown that the mobility practices observed cannot constitute an equitable foundation on which to base the hypotheses for calculating accessibility levels to healthcare. The 2010 Global Transport Survey (EGT, *Enquête Globale Transport*)[9] was used for learning more about the modes of transport used for attending outpatient care in the various Île-de-France areas. It showed that nearly 47% of trips by Parisians towards outpatient care were made on foot, whereas 84% of these were made by private car in rural municipalities in the outer suburbs. However, operational modeling of healthcare accessibility levels calibrated according to these observed modal shares would amount to considering that it is legitimate to regulate the healthcare

9. This survey was carried out under the aegis of the public transport organizing authority in Île-de-France (Île-de-France Mobilités), the Observatory of mobility in Île-de-France (Omnil) and the regional and interdepartmental directorate for Equipment and Urban Planning (DRIEA, *Direction régionale et interdépartementale de l'Équipement et de l'Aménagement*).

provision so that Parisians have a significant supply at their disposal close to their home while the inhabitants of the outer suburbs (including the less mobile and the most confined ones) continue to travel great distances by car.

## 7.7. Rationalization policies take a new direction in France and turn away from mobility

In a very large number of countries in the world, the health system reforms implemented were part of a general process of institutional decentralization. This process prioritized the "local" level to address inequalities in health and was based on the New Public Management[10] logic to redefine operating methods (Eliot et al. 2017). In this way, a new action framework was promoted, leaving more room for actors at the local level to participate in the organization of the health system. It called for more targeted public action on the exploitation of the resources specific to each territory, based on the principle that "patients live and professionals work in the territory, so it is in this very territory that problems and solutions are located" (Clément 2016).

In France, as in England a few years ago (Curtis and Learmonth 2017), there has been an increase in the importance of reorganization policies initiated cooperatively "in the field" alongside rationalization policies stricto sensu. It is the projects and organization of the healthcare actors that must make it possible to foster suitable configurations for organizing the healthcare system at the local level, on a contractual basis between the project promoters and the supervisory authority. This is what is expected from territorial hospital groups (GHT, *Groupements hospitaliers de territoire*) and territorial professional health communities (CPTS, *Communautés professionnelles territoriales de santé*). For both, the goal is to structure the links between local health facilities, on the one hand, and health professionals and social medical actors, on the other hand, as well as to rely on these actors to identify needs and to address local issues.

To some extent, these organizational transformations conceal the concept of mobility in healthcare provision planning, regulation and rationalization policies, in favor of the coordination of relevant actors.

10. For a definition, see Chapoz and Pupion (2012).

## 7.8. Conclusion: limitations of the methods used by the various healthcare rationalization and territorial regulation policies

Significant progress has been made in measuring accessibility to care over the past decade. Alongside traditional density, distance and flow indicators (which remain unavoidable), new measures cross-referencing these indicators make it possible to reconsider former findings (*x*SFCA-type indicators). These advances have been made possible thanks to the development of Geographic Information Systems (GIS) and localized databases, which have refined both the measurement of healthcare supply and demand and the interaction between these dimensions.

However, the search for optimization of the method that will make it possible to prioritize health resource allocation within spaces and populations has been and still remains a long and frustrating process (Ricketts et al. 2007). Regardless of the methodological tools mobilized by the various healthcare rationalization and territorial regulation policies, certain limitations persist.

### 7.8.1. *The geographical entity of reference*

The first of these limitations concerns the choice of the geographical entity for analysis and processing, often done depending on data availability/volume and the processing capacity and/or familiarity of the actors with the breakdown chosen (administrative breakdowns in particular). The adequacy of this geographical entity with the object of analysis is rarely called into question in most countries.

In France, for example, areas with a shortage of general practitioners are defined on the basis of municipal indicators (for ARS methods) or an average of municipal LPA indicators at the “health living territory” level (for the national method). These geographical scales are chosen for pragmatic reasons (databases are available at these scales, processing is not too complex), as well as for operational reasons. Although these are finer scales than the inter-municipal or departmental scales (to respect proximity considerations), their size still grants doctors a sufficient patient base and a coordinated practice, while leaving physicians with a relatively wide choice of settlement locations within vulnerable territories (Vergier and Chaput 2017).

The operational scale thus defined takes precedence over the scale of analysis, but without making adequacy imperatives explicit between the initial scale of analysis and the operational scale. However, research on Île-de-France by Lucas and Mangeney (2019) carried out thanks to the dissemination of data by the administrations and the national statistics services at an infra-municipal level (200-meter grid) showed that the LPA methodology applied at this scale reveals intra-municipal disparities in the access to general practitioners. Furthermore, the 2010 EGT survey indicated that in Île-de-France, nearly a quarter (22%) of journeys towards outpatient care were made less than 500 meters from the place of residence[11], although this figure comprised the recourse to general practitioners and specialists who were known to be more distant. Moreover, since the beginning of the 2000s, reflections on the organization and gradation of the healthcare network considered that access to a general practitioner (pivot and gateway to the care pathway) must be available in “proximity” (Vigneron et al. 2000; Mauss and Polton 2003; Comber et al. 2011; Engels and Liu 2011; HCAM 2017). It is also true that this proximity is not sharply or uniformly defined throughout studies: a few minutes, 5–10 or 20 minutes, 0–5 km from place of residence, etc. (Albe-Tersiguel et al. 2008). However, these elements lead us to think that analyzing the accessibility to general practitioners on a very fine geographical scale would potentially be more consistent with inhabitants’ mobility practices towards healthcare provision.

Thus, we may wonder why the operational territories could not be built from geographically finer analysis indicators that could then be aggregated to reach the critical action size. This remark leads to the following: can the measurement of accessibility to healthcare actually overlook the differences in mobility and needs between individuals?

### 7.8.2. *The specificities of populations*

The second limitation relates to the fact that healthcare accessibility measures often overlook the specificities of populations (in terms of mobility needs and capabilities, in particular). In Belgium, for example, noting that the number of doctors per inhabitant was 30% higher in the part of the

11. This proportion was 32% for Parisians, 24% for the inhabitants of one of the three departments in the inner suburbs, and 15% for the inhabitants of the outer suburbs. If we consider the share of trips towards outpatient care services that took place less than 500 meters from the home or in the municipality of residence, the results were 55% in Paris, 58% in the inner suburbs and 46% in the outer suburbs.

country where the French community lives than where the Flemish community is located, from 2004 the federal government imposed an evolution of the annual quota of graduates in the French community in order to reach an equalization in the number of doctors per inhabitant by 2020 in the two communities of the country (Marchand and Pestieau 2003). Nevertheless, this goal of equalizing medical densities was not accompanied by a reflection on the characteristics and needs of each of the two populations concerned. Even though the healthcare provision planning model was then refined to address care needs according to the different age brackets (Benahmed et al. 2018), the acknowledgment of care need specificities and access modalities to care is still limited.

As far as we know, despite being widely documented (Kaufmann 2008; Vallée et al. 2015) in general, the social differentials in mobility are not often taken into consideration in health planning. Daily mobility is not called into question in relation to the social practices that end up being determined by dispositions and resources unequally distributed in space (Belton-Chevallier et al. 2019). However, from a methodological point of view, some authors (Paez et al. 2010; Engels and Liu 2011) have suggested measuring accessibility levels considering restricted mobility for certain population categories (the elderly without motor vehicles, the poorest populations, etc.) in order to take into account the potentially greater effort these population categories have to make to reach healthcare facilities. It might also be interesting to take into account other accessibility factors making possible the "immobility" of populations (home visits or hospital at home) or facilitating mobility (transport on demand, medical transport, etc.). Is not the failure to take into account the social obstacles to mobility (whether resulting from cognitive cultural dimensions or from temporal or material constraints) in the healthcare rationalization policies a new illustration of the "socio-paresis"[12] mentioned by certain authors (Lombrail et al. 2004)?

### 7.8.3. *A "domo-centric" approach*

Finally, another limitation concerns the nature of the exclusively "domo-centric" character of healthcare rationalization policies, whether

12. Inspired by the words of Jonathan Mann (1998) who described "socio-paresis" as the inability to envisage the social dimension of health problems and denounced the failure of the healthcare system to consider social inequalities in health, ultimately perpetuating or even accentuating them.

based on density, closest distance indicators or derived from gravity models. They do not take into account the different places of activity of individuals (the workplace, places of transit, convenience stores, etc.) and daily mobility practices (see Chapters 1–3). It could be useful to go a step beyond this prioritization of the territories of action depending on the characteristics of the resident populations and to take into account variations in the attributes of these territories throughout the day as well as the potentialities offered to populations in other living territories. In addition, the deficit nature of the residence areas does not have the same implications depending on whether the populations that inhabit them are mobile during the day or not (Vallée 2017).

The main challenge for actors to become familiar with the issues posed by time-geography is the difficulty in statistically getting to know their actual living areas and establishing how individuals use them throughout the day (Kwan 2012a). The development of big data and traveling surveillance via smartphone location can open up new avenues of research in this direction, provided that researchers or decision-makers can complement these data with the demographic and social characteristics of individuals.

The methods developed will also have to take into account the general reorganization of the healthcare system. This is increasingly oriented not only towards coordinated healthcare pathways but also new practices in patient–doctor interaction (telemedicine), which will no longer systematically involve mobility or the co-presence of the specialist and the patient at the same place.

In conclusion, health planning, regulation and rationalization policies are largely based on the measurement of spatial accessibility to care. Following the methodological and technological evolution, the concept of mobility is being increasingly considered in an integrated manner. However, taking mobility into account could still be improved, in particular by adapting the observation scale to the practical scale and differentiating it from the scale of action; by integrating the particular social differentials of mobility and motility and finally, by questioning the timeless and domo-centric nature of mobility, as considered by spatial accessibility. Moreover, the current trend in the reorganization of the healthcare system could potentially relegate the notion of accessibility to the background and favor coordination issues, not to mention the dematerialization of healthcare.

## 7.9. References


Albe-Tersiguel, S., Blum, E., de Berny Riche, C., Delaporte, C., Mangeney, C., Parnaix, A., Peuvergne C. (2008). Démarche exploratoire pour une hiérarchisation des équipements en Île-de-France. Report, Institut Paris Région, Paris.

Allan, D. (2014). Catchments of general practice in different countries – A literature review. *International Journal of Health Geographics*, 13, 32.

Apparicio, P., Abdelmajid, M., Riva, M., Shearmur, R. (2008). Comparing alternative approaches to measuring the geographical accessibility of urban health services: Distance types and aggregation-error issues. *International Journal of Health Geographics*, 7(1), 7.

Aschan-Leygonie, C. (2017). Des solutions pour améliorer l'accessibilité aux soins : l'expérience suédoise. *Revue francophone sur la santé et les territoires*. doi: 10.4000/rfst.597.

Bacqué, M.H. and Fol, S. (2007). L'inégalité face à la mobilité : du constat à l'injonction. *Revue suisse de sociologie*, 33(1), 89.

Bailoni, M. (2011). Les inégalités territoriales et les enjeux géopolitiques de la santé au Royaume-Uni. *Herodote*, 143(4), 162–183.

Barer, M.L. and Stoddart, G.L. (1992). Toward integrated medical resource policies for Canada: 8. Geographic distribution of physicians. *Canadian Medical Association Journal*, 147(5), 617–623.

Barlet, M., Coldefy, M., Collin, C., Lucas-Gabrielli, V. (2012). L'accessibilité potentielle localisée (APL) : une nouvelle mesure de l'accessibilité aux soins appliquée aux médecins généralistes libéraux en France. Report, Institut de recherche et documentation en économie de la santé, Paris.

Bavoux, J.J. and Chapelon, L. (2015). *Dictionnaire d'analyse spatiale*. Armand Colin, Paris.

Belton-Chevallier, L., Oppenchaim, N., Vincent-Geslin, S. (2019). *Manuel de sociologie des mobilités géographiques*. Presses Universitaires François Rabelais, Tours.

Benahmed, N., Deliège, B., De Wever, A., Pirson, M. (2018). La planification des médecins en Europe : une revue de la littérature des modèles de projection. *Revue d'Épidémiologie et de Santé Publique*, 66, 63–73.

Bonerandi, E. (2004). De la mobilité en géographie. *Géoconfluences* [Online]. Available at: http://geoconfluences.ens-lyon.fr/doc/transv/Mobil/MobilScient.htm.

Bouleau, M. and Mangeney, C. (2015). Déplacements et usages de la métropole. Coupes et découpes territoriales – quelles réalité du Bassin de vie ? *Les Cahiers IAU-IdF*, 172, 81–86.

Bourgueil, Y., Tajahmadi, A., Mousques, J. (2006). Comment améliorer la répartition géographique des professionnels de santé ? Les enseignements de la littérature internationale et des mesures adoptées en France. Report, IRDES, Paris.

Brunet, R. (1997). Territoires : l'art de la découpe/Pinking shears applied to territories. *Géocarrefour*, 72(3), 251–255.

Carr-Hill, R., Place, M., Possnett, J. (1997). Access and the utilisation of healthcare services. In *Concentration and Choice in Healthcare*, Ferguson, B., Sheldon, T., Posnett, J. (eds). Financial Times Healthcare, London.

Chappoz, Y. and Pupion, P.C. (2012). Le new public management. *Gestion et management public*, 1/2(2), 1–3.

Chardonnel, S. (2007). Time-geography: Individuals in time and space. In *Models in Spatial Analysis*, Sanders, L. (ed.). ISTE Ltd, London, and John Wiley & Sons, New York.

Charreire, H., Casey, R., Salze, P., Simon, C., Banos, A., Badariotti, D., Weber, C., Oppert, J.M. (2010). Measuring the food environment using geographical information systems: A methodological review. *Public Health Nutrition*, 13(11), 1773–1785.

Charron, M. and Shearmur, R. (2005). Distances, interactions et analyse spatiale de la ville : le cas de Montréal. *Revue d'Économie Régionale et Urbaine*, 2, 163–192.

Cheng, J. and Bertolini, L. (2013). Measuring urban job accessibility with distance decay, competition and diversity. *Journal of Transport Geography*, 30, 100–109.

Chevallier, J. (2004). L'état régulateur. *Revue française d'administration publique*, 3(111), 473–482.

Clément, J.M. (2016). *La loi santé 2016 : analyse, commentaires, critiques.* Les Études Hospitalières Édition, Bordeaux.

Coldefy, M. and Lefebvre, B. (2019). *Abécédaire de la géographie de la santé. Dimension territoriale de la santé*. Éditions Matériologiques, Paris.

Coldefy, M. and Lucas-Gabrielli, V. (2010). Les territoires de santé : des approches régionales variées de ce nouvel espace de planification. *Pratiques et Organisation des Soins*, 41(1), 73.

Comber, A.J., Brunsdon, C., Radburn, R. (2011). A spatial analysis of variations in health access: Linking geography, socio-economic status and access perceptions. *International Journal of Health Geographics*, 10(1), 44.

Cromley, E.K. and McLafferty, S.L. (2002). *GIS and Public Health*. Guilford Press, New York.

Curtis, S. and Learmonth, A. (2017). La décentralisation va-t-elle améliorer la santé et réduire les inégalités de santé au Royaume-Uni ? *Revue francophone sur la santé et les territoires*. doi: 10.4000/rfst.586.

Dagorn, C., Giorgi, D., Meunier, A. (2019). Bilan d'étape des groupements hospitaliers de territoires (GHT). Report, IGAS, 2019-034R, 129.

Dai, D. and Wang, F. (2011). Geographic disparities in accessibility to food stores in south-west Mississippi. *Environment and Planning B: Planning and Design*, 38, 659–677.

Delamater, P. (2013). Spatial accessibility in suboptimally configured health care systems: A modified two-step floating catchment area (M2SFCA) metric. *Health & Place*, 24, 30–43.

Eliot, E., Lucas-Gabrielli, V., Mangeney, C. (2017). Territorialisation sanitaire et décentralisation : état des lieux et enjeux à partir du cas français. *Revue francophone sur la santé et les territoires*. doi: 10.4000/rfst.577.

Ellegård, K. and Svedin, U. (2012). Torsten Hägerstrand's time-geography as the cradle of the activity approach in transport geography. *Journal of Transport Geography*, 23, 17–25.

Engels, B. and Liu, G.J. (2011). Social exclusion, location and transport disadvantage amongst non-driving seniors in a Melbourne municipality. *Journal of Transport Geography*, 19(4), 984–996.

European Observatory on Health Systems and Policies (2020). Health system reviews (HiT series). WHO, Geneva.

Fol, S. and Gallez, C. (2013). Mobilité, accessibilité et équité : pour un renouvellement de l'analyse des inégalités sociales d'accès à la ville. *Colloque International Futurs urbains : Enjeux interdisciplinaires émergents pour comprendre, projeter et fabriquer la ville de demain*, Champs-sur-Marne [Online]. Available at: https://shs.hal.science/halshs-00780292/document.

Forzy, L., Titli, L., Carpezat, M. (2021). Accès aux soins et pratiques de recours, étude sur le vécu des patients. *Les dossiers de la DREES*, 77.

Geurs, K.T. and Van Wee, B. (2004). Accessibility evaluation of land-use and transport strategies: Review and research directions. *Journal of Transport Geography*, 12(2), 127–140.

Gould, P. and Leinbach, T.R. (1966). An approach to the geographic assignment of hospital services. *Tijdschrift voor Economische en Sociale Geographie*, 57, 203–206.

Hägerstrand, T. (1970). What about people in Regional Science? *Regional Science Association Papers*, XXIV.

Handy, S.L. and Niemeier, D.A. (1997). Measuring accessibility: An exploration of issues and alternatives. *Environment and Planning A*, 29(7), 1175–1194.

Hassenteufel, P., Schweyer, F.-X., Gerlinger, T., Reiter, R. (2020). Les "déserts médicaux" comme leviers de la réorganisation des soins primaires, une comparaison entre la France et l'Allemagne. *Revue française des affaires sociales*, 33–56.

Hays, S.M., Kearns, R.A., Moran, W. (1990). Spatial patterns of attendance at general practitioner services. *Social Sciences and Medicine*, 31(7), 773–791.

HCAM (2017). Médecine spécialisée et organisation des soins : les spécialistes dans l'offre de soins, séance du 23 mars 2017. Report.

Hunter, J.M., Shannon, G.W., Sambrook, S.L. (1986). Rings of madness: Service areas of 19th century asylums in North America. *Social Science and Medicine*, 23(10), 1033–1050.

Jamtsho, S., Corner, R., Dewan, A. (2015). Spatio-temporal analysis of spatial accessibility to primary health care in Bhutan. *ISPRS International Journal of Geo-Information*, 4(3), 1584–1604.

Joseph, A.E. and Phillips, D.R. (1984). *Accessibility and Utilization: Geographical Perspectives on Health Care Delivery*. Harper, New York.

Julien, P. (2004). La France en 1916 bassins de vie. *Economie et statistique*, 402, 25–39.

Kaufman, V. (2001). La motilité : une notion clé pour revisiter l'urbain ? In *Enjeux de la sociologie urbaine*, Bassand, M., Kaufmann, V., Joye, D. (eds). Presses polytechniques et universitaires romandes, Lausanne.

Kaufmann, V. (2008). *Les paradoxes de la mobilité, bouger, s'enraciner*. Presses polytechniques et universitaires romandes, Lausanne.

de Kervasdoué, J. and Picheral, H. (2004). *Santé et territoire. Carnet de santé de la France*. Dunod, Paris.

Kwan, M. (2004). GIS methods in time-geographic research: Geocomputation and geovisualization of human activity patterns. *Geografiska Annaler: Series B, Human Geography*, 86(4), 267–280.

Lacoste, O. and Spinosi, L. (2002). Distance, proximité, accessibilité, attraction et recours de la population vis-à-vis du système de soins. Report, Observatoire régional de la santé (ORS), Paris.

Langford, M., Higgs, G., Fry, R. (2016). Multi-modal two-step floating catchment area analysis of primary health care accessibility. *Health & Place*, 38, 70–81.

Lévy, J. and Lussault, M. (2013). *Dictionnaire de la géographie et de l'espace des sociétés*. Belin, Paris.

Li, Z., Serban, N., Swann, J.L. (2015). An optimization framework for measuring spatial access over healthcare networks. *BMC Health Services Research*, 15(1), 273.

Lombrail, P., Lang, T., Pascal, J. (2004). Accès au système de soins et inégalités sociales de santé : que sait-on de l'accès secondaire ? *Santé, Société et Solidarité*, 3(2), 61–71.

Lucas-Gabrielli, V. and Mangeney, C. (2019). L'accessibilité aux médecins généralistes en Île-de-France : méthodologie de mesures des inégalités infra-communales. Working paper, 80.

Lucas-Gabrielli, V., Pierre, A., Com-Ruelle, L., Coldefy, M. (2016). *Pratiques spatiales d'accès aux soins*. IRDES, Paris.

Luo, J. (2014). Integrating the huff model and floating catchment area methods to analyze spatial access to healthcare services. *Transactions in GIS*, 18(3), 436–448.

Luo, W. and Wang, F. (2003). Measures of spatial accessibility to health care in a GIS environment: Synthesis and a case study in the Chicago region. *Environment and Planning B: Planning and Design ER*, 30.

Luo, W. and Whippo, T. (2012). Variable catchment sizes for the two-step floating catchment area (2SFCA) method. *Health & Place*, 18, 789–795.

Macé, J.M. (2002). Une méthode pour définir des "bassins d'hospitalisation" en Ile-de-France. *INSEE*, 209.

Mao, L. and Nekorchuk, D. (2013). Measuring spatial accessibility to healthcare for populations with multiple transportation modes. *Health & Place*, 24, 115–122.

Marchand, M. and Pestieau, P. (2003). Le numerus clausus en médecine : pourquoi et comment ? *Reflets et perspectives de la vie economique*, XLII(1), 59–70.

Mathian, H. and Sanders, L. (2006). Scientific approach of the MAUP? Report, ESPON 3.4.3, ESPON 2000-2006 program, 1–33.

Mauss, H. and Polton, D. (2003). Territoires et accès aux soins. Report, La Documentation française, Paris

McGrail, M.R. (2012). Spatial accessibility of primary health care utilising the two step floating catchment area method: An assessment of recent improvements. *International Journal of Health Geographics*, 11(1), 50.

McGrail, M.R. and Humphreys, J.S. (2009a). A new index of access to primary care services in rural areas. *Australian and New Zealand Journal of Public Health*, 33(5), 418–423.

McGrail, M.R. and Humphreys, J.S. (2009b). Measuring spatial accessibility to primary care in rural areas: Improving the effectiveness of the two-step floating catchment area method. *Applied Geography*, 29(4), 533–541.

McGrail, M.R. and Humphreys, J.S. (2009c). The index of rural access: An innovative integrated approach for measuring primary care access. *BMC Health Services Research*, 9(1), 124.

McGrail, M.R. and Humphreys, J.S. (2014). Measuring spatial accessibility to primary health care services: Utilising dynamic catchment sizes. *Applied Geography*, 54, 182–188.

Meade, M.S. and Earickson, R.J. (2000). *Medical Geography*, 2nd edition. Guilford Press, New York.

Merlin, P. and Choay, F. (2010). *Dictionnaire de l'urbanisme et de l'aménagement*. PUF, Paris.

Missinne, S. and Luyten, S. (2018). Les médecins généralistes en région bruxelloise : qui sont-ils, où pratiquent-ils et où se situent les potentielles pénuries ? Report, Observatoire de la Santé et du Social/Commission communautaire commune, Brussels.

Mizrahi, A. and Mizrahi, A. (2010). La densité répartie : un instrument de mesure des inégalités géographiques d'accès aux soins. *Villes en parallèle*, 44(1), 94–113.

Morrill, R.L. and Earickson, R. (1969). Locational efficiency of Chicago hospitals: An experimental model. *Health Services Research*, 4(2), 128–141.

Neutens, T. (2015). Accessibility, equity and health care: Review and research directions for transport geographers. *Journal of Transport Geography*, 43.

OECD (2016). Health Workforce Policies in OECD Countries: Right Jobs, Right Skills, Right Places.

Openshaw, S. (1984). Ecological fallacies and the analysis of areal census data. *Environment and Planning A*, 16, 17–31.

Paez, A., Mercado, R.G., Farber, S., Morency, C., Roorda, M. (2010). Accessibility to health care facilities in Montreal Island: An application of relative accessibility indicators from the perspective of senior and non-senior residents. *International Journal of Health Geographics*, 9(1), 52.

Palier, B. (2017). *La réforme des systèmes de santé.* Presses Universitaires de France, Paris.

Peng, Z.R. (1997). The jobs-housing balance and urban commuting. *Urban Studies*, 34(8), 1215–1235.

Picheral, H. (2001). *Dictionnaire raisonné de géographie de la santé.* Université Montpellier III, Montpellier.

Radke, J. and Mu, L. (2000). Spatial decompositions, modeling and mapping service regions to predict access to social programs. *Annals of GIS*, 6, 105–112.

Rican, S. and Vaillant, Z. (2009). Territoires et santé : enjeux sanitaires de la territorialisation et enjeux territoriaux des politiques de santé. *Sciences sociales et santé*, 27(1), 33–42.

Ricketts, T. (2010). Accessing health care. In *A Companion to Health and Medical Geography*, Brown, T. and Moon, G. (eds). Wiley-Blackwell, Hoboken.

Ricketts, T., Goldsmith, L., Holmes, M., Randolph, R., Lee, R., Taylor, D., Ostermann, J. (2007). Designating places and populations as medically underserved: A proposal for a new approach. *Journal of Health Care for the Poor and Underserved*, 18, 567–589.

Rosenberg, M.W. (1988). Linking the gegraphical, the medical and the political in analyzing health care delivery systems. *Social Science and Medicine*, 26.

Salze, P., Banos, A., Oppert, J.M. (2011). Estimating spatial accessibility to facilities on the regional scale: An extended commuting-based interaction potential model. *International Journal of Health Geographics*, 10(2).

Talen, E. and Anselin, L. (1998). Assessing spatial equity: An evaluation of measures of accessibility to public playgrounds. *Environment and Planning A: Economy and Space*, 30(4), 595–613.

Tao, Z., Cheng, Y., Zheng, Q., Li, G. (2018). Measuring spatial accessibility to healthcare services with constraint of administrative boundary: A case study of Yanqing District, Beijing, China. *International Journal for Equity in Health*, 17(1), 7.

Thouez, J.P. (1987). *Organisation spatiale des systèmes de soins*. Les Presses de l'Université de Montréal, Montreal.

Vallée, J. (2017). Challenges in targeting areas for public action. Target areas at the right place and at the right time. *Journal of Epidemiology and Community Health*, 71(10), 945.

Vallée, J., Commenges, H., Perchoux, C., Kestens, Y., Chaix, B. (2015). Mobilité quotidienne et accès potentiel aux ressources urbaines : quelles inégalités sociales ? *Données urbaines* 7, 87–95.

Vergier, N. and Chaput, H. (2017). Déserts médicaux : comment les définir ? Comment les mesurer ? *Les dossiers de la DREES*, 17.

Vigneron, E. and Brau, F. (1996). Approches géographiques de la planification sanitaire : concepts et méthodes. *Cahiers GEOS*, 32.

Vigneron, E. and Corvez, A. (1999). Santé publique et aménagement du territoire. *Actualité et dossier en santé publique*, 29.

Vigneron, E., Glatron M., Jacob, J.Y. (2000). Santé publique et aménagement du territoire. *Actes du Festival international de géographie de Saint-Dié des Vosges*.

Wan, N., Zou, B., Sternberg, T. (2012). A three-step floating catchment area method for analyzing spatial access to health services. *International Journal of Geographical Information Science*, 26(6), 1073–1089.

Wang, F. (2012). Measurement, optimization, and impact of health care accessibility: A methodological review. *Annals of the Association of American Geographers*, 102(5), 1104–1112.

Wang, F. and Luo, W. (2005). Assessing spatial and nonspatial factors for healthcare access: Towards an integrated approach to defining health professional shortage areas. *Heath and Place*, 11(2), 131–146.

# List of Authors

Stephanie ALEXANDER
Fondation d'entreprise MGEN
pour la santé publique
Paris
France

Alexandre CEBEILLAC
IDEES, CNRS
Normandie Université
Rouen
and
Institut Pasteur
Paris
France

Hélène CHARREIRE
MoISA
Cirad
CIHEAM-IAMM
INRAE
Institut Agro
IRD
Université de Montpellier
and
Lab'URBA
Université Paris-Est Créteil
and
Institut universitaire de France
Paris
France

Marie-Soleil CLOUTIER
LAPS
Institut national de la
recherche scientifique
Montreal
Canada

Eric DAUDÉ
IDEES, CNRS
Normandie Université
Rouen
France

Thierry FEUILLET
IDEES
Université de Caen
and
EREN
Université Sorbonne Paris Nord
Bobigny
France

Karine LACHAPELLE
LAPS
Institut national de la recherche scientifique
Montreal
Canada

Véronique LUCAS-GABRIELLI
Irdes
Paris
France

Catherine MANGENEY
ORS Île-de-France
Paris
and
Géographie-cités
Université Paris Cité
France

Camille PERCHOUX
LISER
Esch-sur-Alzette
Luxembourg

Martine SHARECK
Université de Sherbrooke
Canada

Julie VALLÉE
Géographie-cités
CNRS
Paris
France

# Index

**G, H**



**I, L**



**M, N**



**O, P**



**Q, R**



**S, T**

## V, W

Printed and bound by CPI Group (UK) Ltd, Croydon, CR0 4YY
13/09/2026
14960998-0001